American Grown

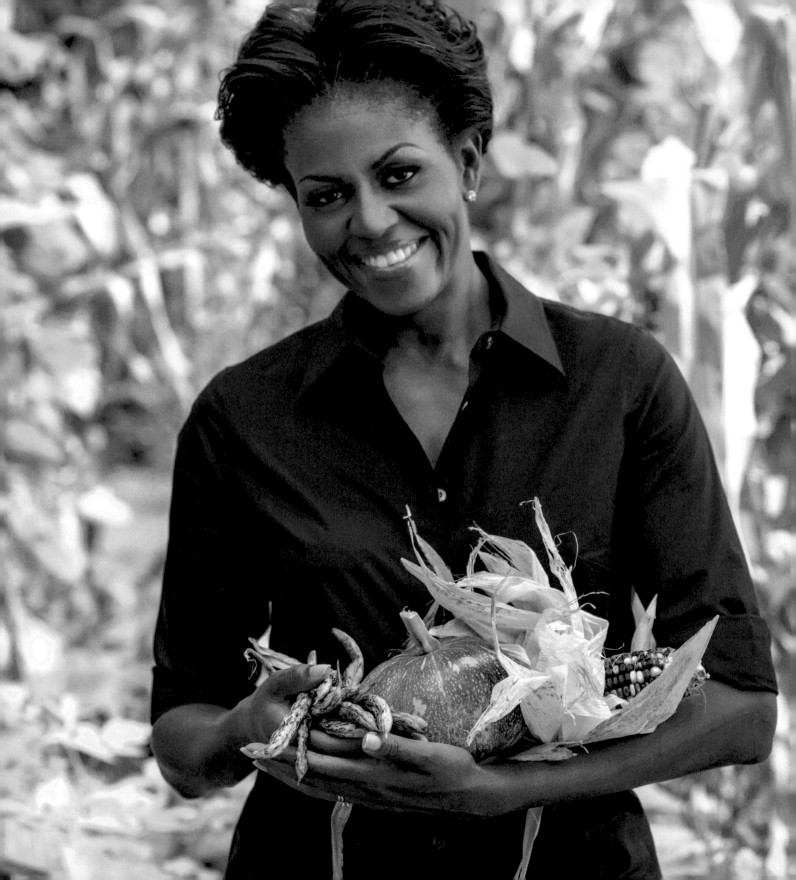

American Grown

The Story of the White House Kitchen Garden and Gardens Across America

Michelle Obama

CROWN PUBLISHERS
New York

Copyright © 2012 by the National Park Foundation

All rights reserved.
Published in the United States by Crown Publishers,
an imprint of the Crown Publishing Group,
a division of Random House, Inc., New York.
www.crownpublishing.com

CROWN and the Crown colophon are registered
trademarks of Random House, Inc.

Photo credits appear on page 267.

Library of Congress Cataloging-in-Publication Data is
available upon request

ISBN 978-0-307-95602-6
eISBN 978-0-307-95603-3

Printed in the United States of America

Book design by Marysarah Quinn
Original illustrations, garden plans, and endpaper art by Ken Krug
Jacket design by Marysarah Quinn
Jacket photographs by Quentin Bacon Photography

10 9 8 7 6 5 4 3 2 1

First Edition

To all the gardeners, farmers, educators, advocates,
community leaders, parents, and others who have been
leading the way for years, teaching us about the food we
grow and the impact it has on our families' health.

To our nation's children, who deserve to grow up healthy
and strong and have every chance to pursue their dreams.

And to my husband and daughters for their boundless love
and countless hours of conversation around the dinner
table—you are the center of my world, and I could not have
done this without you.

Contents

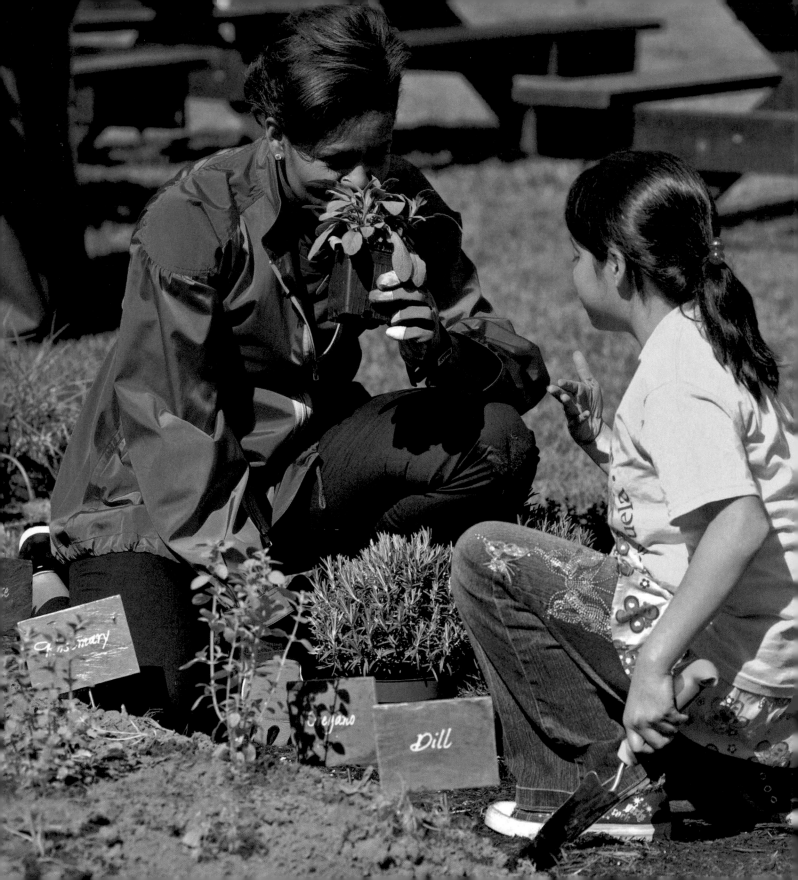

INTRODUCTION

On March 20, 2009, I was like any other hopeful gardener with a pot out on the windowsill or a small plot by the back door. I was nervously watching the sky. Would it freeze? Would it snow? Would it rain? I had spent two months settling into a new house in a new city. My girls had started a new school; my husband, a new job. My mother had just moved in upstairs. And now I was embarking on something I had never attempted before: starting a garden.

But this was not going to be just any garden—it would be a very public garden. Cameras would be trained on its beds, and questions would be asked about what we had planted and why we had planted it. The garden was also being planted on a historic landscape: the South Lawn of the White House. Here even the tomatoes and beans would have a view of the towering Washington Monument.

When I first arrived in Washington, I wasn't even sure that we could plant a garden. I didn't know whether we would be allowed to change the landscaping on the White House grounds, or whether the soil would be fertile enough, or whether there would be enough sunlight. And I had hardly any gardening experience, so I didn't even really know how to go about planting a garden in the first place.

But one thing I did know was that I wanted this garden to be more than just a plot of land growing vegetables on the White House lawn. I wanted it to be the starting point for something bigger. As both a mother and a first lady, I was alarmed by reports of skyrocketing childhood obesity rates and the dire consequences for our children's health. And I hoped this garden would help begin a conversation about this issue—a conversation about the food we eat, the lives we lead, and how all of that affects our children.

OUR FIRST PLANTING DAY,
APRIL 9, 2009
Our first Kitchen Garden comes to life on planting day, with seedlings, shovels, sunshine, freshly turned soil, and a vision of all that could grow here.

I also knew that I wanted this new White House garden to be a "learning garden," a place where people could have a hands-on experience of working the soil and children who have never seen a plant sprout could put down seeds and seedlings that would take root. And I wanted them to come back for the harvest, to be able to see and taste the fruits (and vegetables) of their labors.

So in 2009, on a chilly and windy, but thankfully sunny, first day of spring, I joined twenty-three fifth graders from Bancroft Elementary School in Washington, D.C., with shovels, rakes, pitchforks, and a few wheelbarrows to break ground for the White House Kitchen Garden. Twenty days later, we were ready to plant. We put in lettuce and peas, spinach and broccoli, kale and collard greens. And for days after that, I would look at the freshly turned soil and wonder to myself, is anything growing?

GROUNDBREAKING,
MARCH 20, 2009
I scooped up layers of history as we broke ground for the garden on the South Lawn of the White House with the help of students from Bancroft Elementary School in Washington, D.C. Bancroft students returned a few weeks later to help plant the new garden space.

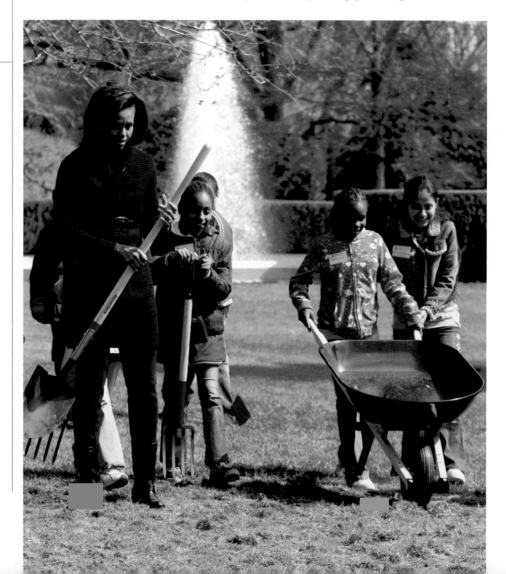

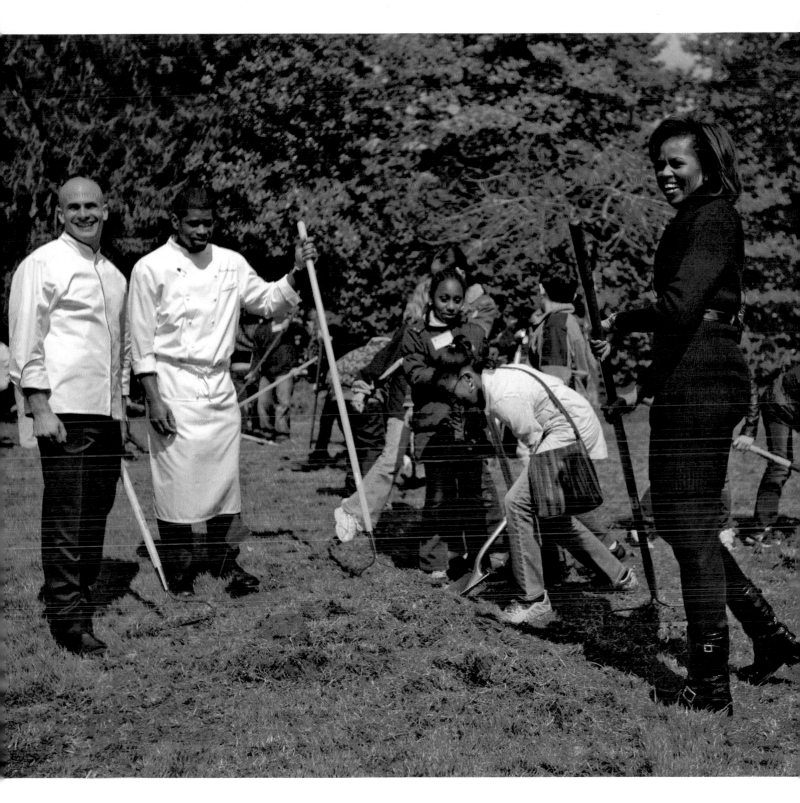

Uncovering My Roots

Like many American schoolkids, as a child, I came home one spring afternoon with a seed that had sprouted in a paper cup. But vegetable gardening wasn't exactly a common pastime in the neighborhood where I grew up, at least not by the time I came along.

I was raised on the South Side of Chicago, the part of the city that backs up to Lake Michigan and stretches all the way out to the Indiana border, as were both my parents.

My mother came from a large family, and in her home someone was always cooking something to feed all the children. They often used fresh ingredients from the vegetable truck that would come around selling produce, much of it straight from the farm. My father actually worked on one of those trucks as a boy, and every time the vegetable man looked up, he would see my father sneaking a piece of fruit, or so the story goes.

VEGETABLE TRUCK
One of the early Chicago fruit and vegetable trucks, which served as an easy, affordable way to get produce to urban neighborhoods. My father worked on one of the trucks and particularly loved to eat the fruit.

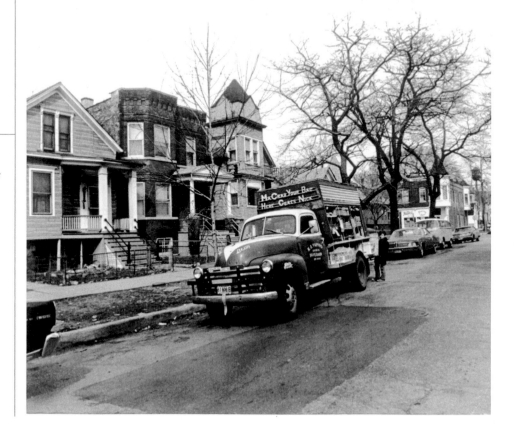

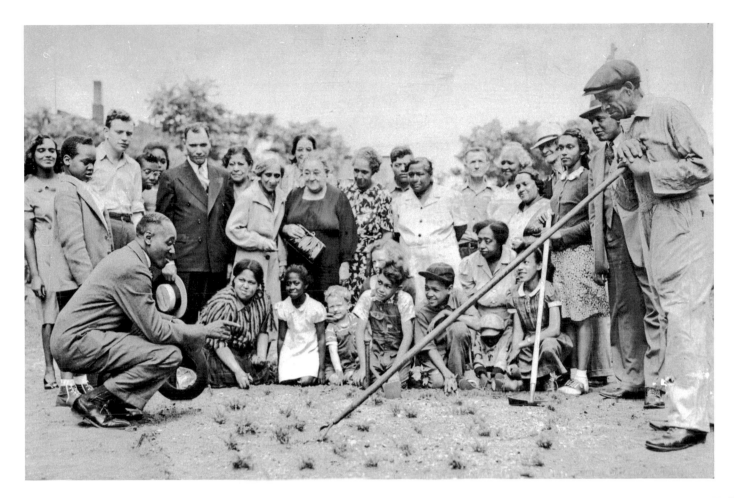

When my mother was a little girl of five or six—around the beginning of World War II—her family had a plot in a local victory garden. On the corner of an alley near her home, a vacant lot had been turned into plots for each family in the neighborhood, and my mother used to accompany her own mother to tend it. They grew corn, tomatoes, green beans, peas, and spinach from seed packets. The children in her family ate their vegetables, whether they liked them or not; otherwise they went to bed without supper.

By the time my mother was grown and married, and my brother and I had come along, nearly all the victory gardens were gone. So were the vegetable trucks. Instead, we ate supermarket produce, picked up when my mother made her weekly trek to buy groceries. My mother made iceberg lettuce salads and cooked broccoli, peas, and carrots along with spaghetti and meatballs or lemon chicken. Over time she branched out and sautéed

VICTORY GARDEN
During World War II, Chicago led the nation in growing victory gardens. The city had some 1,500 community gardens and more than 250,000 home gardens under cultivation. Above, a photograph of Chicago victory gardeners in 1942.

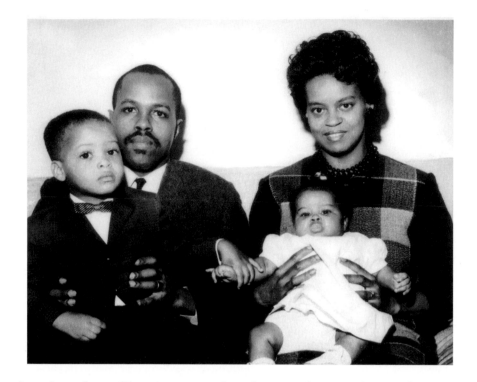

a lot of zucchini. But no matter what she served, every dinner featured at least one vegetable. And we had to eat all of it, no exceptions. Dessert was a treat for Sundays, and most lunches were a sandwich made from last night's leftovers. Our apartment didn't have a dining room, so we ate at the kitchen table. And unless my dad was working the evening shift at his job at the city water plant, we ate our meals together as a family, a tradition that Barack and I have continued with our own children.

It was a good thing my mother made us all those nutritious meals, because back then, we were always in motion. Most kids walked to school every day, rain or shine. I can still remember how when I was very little—maybe three or four years old—my mother and I would go to our gate each morning and watch my older brother, Craig, head off to school. I couldn't wait for the day when I too could venture down the street with a backpack and brown bag lunch. As the years passed, my brother's walk home sometimes became an athletic activity of its own. He was very cute, and I'll never forget seeing him running around the corner, being chased by a pack of screaming girls.

Once we arrived at school, we'd run around on the playground until the bell rang. We had recess every day and gym class every week, and after school we'd head home to our neighborhood and play outside for hours. There were always plenty of kids around, and we'd play softball or a game called Piggy with a batter, a pitcher, a catcher, and a sixteen-inch softball rather than the standard twelve-inch ones (a lot of things are a little bigger in Chicago). The goal was to catch the batter's ball off one bounce or on the fly, so the pitcher or catcher could change places and become the batter. Later, we played chase, which was basically just boys chasing girls and then girls chasing boys. And all the girls in the neighborhood knew how to jump Double Dutch. We would also hop on our bikes and ride around for hours. I still remember when I was finally old enough to ride my bicycle around the sidewalks of the entire block, just like my big brother. It was especially exciting to ride through the alley behind our house. It was dark and filled with shadows that made all the houses look spookier as we raced past them.

As I grew older, I was allowed to venture farther away from our street on my bike. One of my first big solo rides was twenty city blocks to Rainbow Beach Park, home of Rocky Ledge Beach along Lake Michigan, where I could walk along the rocks way out into the lake and have a beautiful view of the city. Often, when I went there, I would pick up friends on their own bikes along the way and we'd ride together. In the summers, I would don my white Chicago Park District camp shirt and head off to day camp at Rainbow Beach, where campers from around the city would come together at the end of the summer for a big Olympics competition.

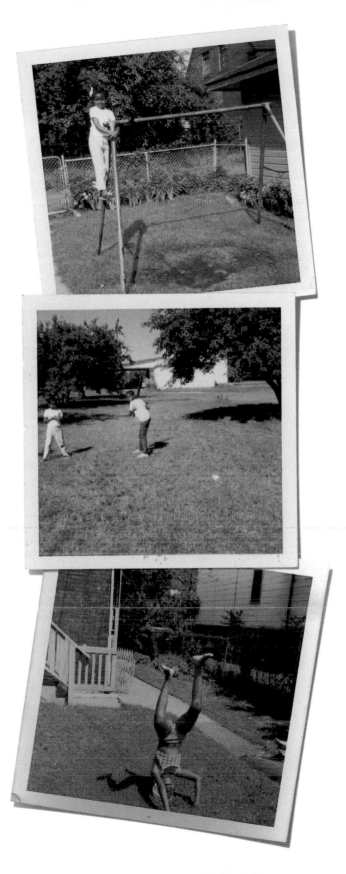

How Times Have Changed

Life in my old neighborhood has changed a great deal since I was young. At my old elementary school, as in many others across America, outdoor recess has been eliminated, and many kids no longer walk to school. While my parents never thought twice about sending us outside to play, parents in that neighborhood today worry about letting their kids venture too far out of their sight. And kids there, like everywhere these days, are probably a lot more likely to huddle around a video game console than join in a game of Double Dutch.

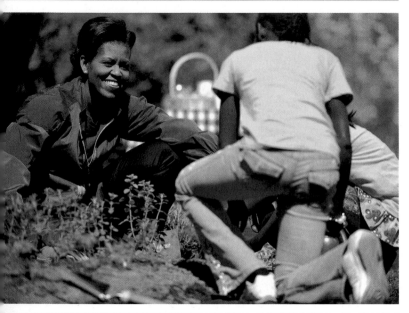

Parents today are squeezed from every direction, always racing to the next appointment, the next carpool pickup, the next errand on their lists. I've been one of those mothers, anxiously looking at my watch while waiting in the drive-through lane or popping something into the microwave while finishing up a conference call.

But I had never really thought about the consequences until I sat down with our family pediatrician, and he asked me a simple question: What are you eating? He then started telling me about how some families in his practice ate every meal—breakfast, lunch, and dinner—at a different convenience-food chain. Aside from a piece of pickle or a sprinkle of shredded lettuce on a hamburger, they had hardly any fruits and vegetables in their diets. He talked about the spike in the number of his young patients who were overweight or even obese. He spoke of kids around the country who are developing adult "lifestyle" diseases: elementary school students being diagnosed with type 2 diabetes and high schoolers already on blood pressure medication. In recent years, the problem has only gotten worse, and today roughly one in three American children are overweight or obese.

That moment was a wake-up call for me. Until then, I thought my husband and I were doing everything we could to give our daughters every opportunity in their lives. We read to them and made sure they did their homework. We signed them up for sports, music lessons, and dance classes.

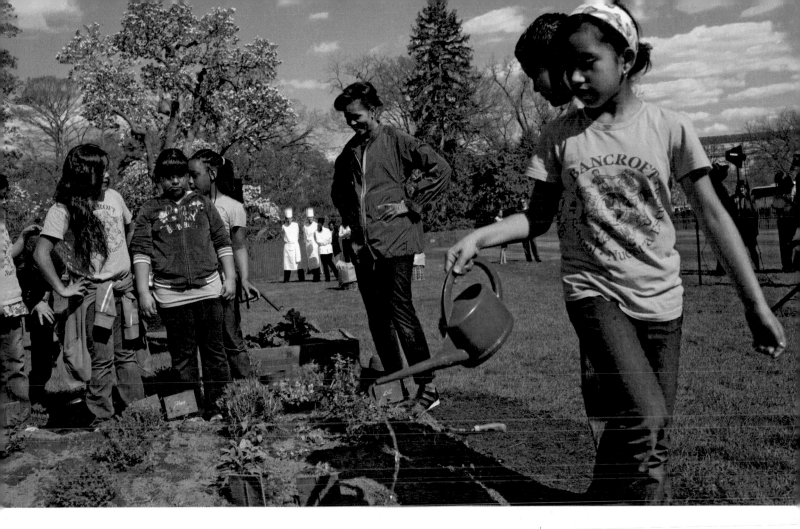

But after talking with their doctor, I realized that we weren't giving them one of the most fundamental advantages they could have: a truly healthy lifestyle.

So we decided to make some changes. We started small, emptying our pantry of unhealthy foods and filling our glasses with water and skim milk instead of sugary drinks. We ate at home more often. We began to add more vegetables to our meals. We discovered farmers' markets and locally grown, fresh produce. And desserts became a treat for the weekends.

Soon we all began to feel better. We were more alert during the day, slept better at night, and had more energy. We got more pleasure out of our meals, and my girls had fun learning about where their food came from. Having information about, and access to, fresh, healthy foods—particularly fruits and vegetables—had a real impact on our health.

OUR FIRST PLANTING DAY,
APRIL 9, 2009

With a gentle shower of water, our first-ever Kitchen Garden plants are ready to grow on the White House's South Lawn.

How Our Gardens Can Help

Some of the changes we've seen in kids' lives over the years are inevitable. Times change, and we can't turn back the clock to the days when the vegetable truck rolled down the street (although there are some twenty-first-century vegetable trucks on a few of our city streets today). But regardless of how the world may change around us, we still have the power to make good choices about what we feed our families. And gardens across the country are playing a vital role in that process.

So I had high hopes for those tiny seeds and seedlings going into the grounds of the White House on that spring morning back in 2009. I knew that growing a garden wouldn't be easy. As farmers can tell you, too much or too little rain, a bad freeze, or a storm at just the wrong time can ruin a crop in a few hours or even a few minutes. Some things that get planted just won't grow, and others grow far too well, taking over the garden. But whatever detours or bumps in the road we would face, I was determined that this garden would succeed.

Fortunately, it did. The seeds took root; the plants grew and produced all kinds of fruits and vegetables; and each new season in our garden brought new gifts and lessons. Spring was a time for new beginnings, when we would plant the seeds of what we hoped to harvest for the rest of the year. Summer was a season of rapid, often breathtaking growth, with plants shooting up and new fruits and vegetables ripening every day. The bounty of fall taught us how, by investing ourselves—our time, energy, and love—we were able to fulfill the promise of spring and share our harvest with others. During the winter, we learned that with a little imagination and a lot of hard work, we could extend the life of our garden beyond what we ever thought possible.

FALL HARVEST DAY 2009
The giant sweet potatoes were an unexpected surprise. Everyone wanted to dig up a potato. And they tasted great!

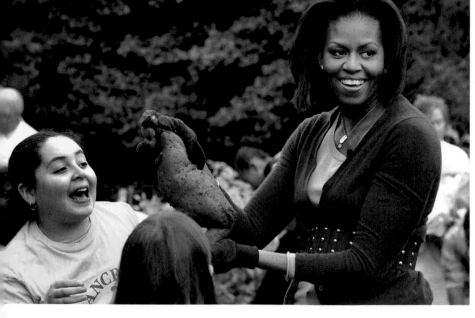

And over the past three years, our White House Kitchen Garden has bloomed into so much more. It's helped us start a new conversation about the food we eat and how it affects our children's health. It's helped us raise awareness about our crisis of childhood obesity and the threat it poses to our children's future. And it led to the creation of *Let's Move!,* a nationwide initiative to solve this problem so our children can grow up healthy.

This book tells that story. In it you'll learn about how we designed and planted our garden and all the children, volunteers, and staff members who plant, tend, and harvest it. We also provide tips on how to start your own garden and how to prepare and store the fruits and vegetables you grow and buy. And we include original recipes from the White House chefs to help you put them to good use preparing fresh, delicious meals and snacks for yourself and your family.

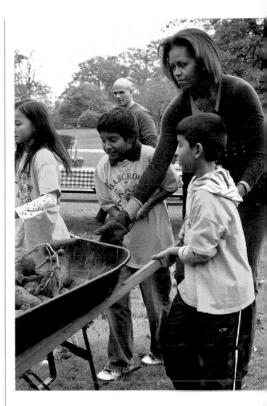

But the purpose of this book is not simply to share our own story. Our White House Kitchen Garden is just one of thousands of gardens across this country, each with a story worth telling. In my hometown of Chicago, there's a World War II victory garden that still blooms today. In Houston, Texas, there's a garden adjacent to a downtown building where office workers tend to okra, squash, and tomatoes planted in containers on the concrete sidewalk. Teachers, parents, and students have started school gardens. Neighborhood gardeners are growing crops for local food banks. And people from all walks of life and every sector of our society are coming together and using gardens—and the food they grow and lessons they teach—to build a healthier future for our children.

It is my hope that our garden's story—and the stories of gardens across America—will inspire families, schools, and communities to try their own hand at gardening and enjoy all the gifts of health, discovery, and connection a garden can bring.

All across this great country of ours, something truly special is taking root. And that is the story I want to tell in this book: the story of how, together, in gardens large and small, we have begun to grow a healthier nation.

Spring

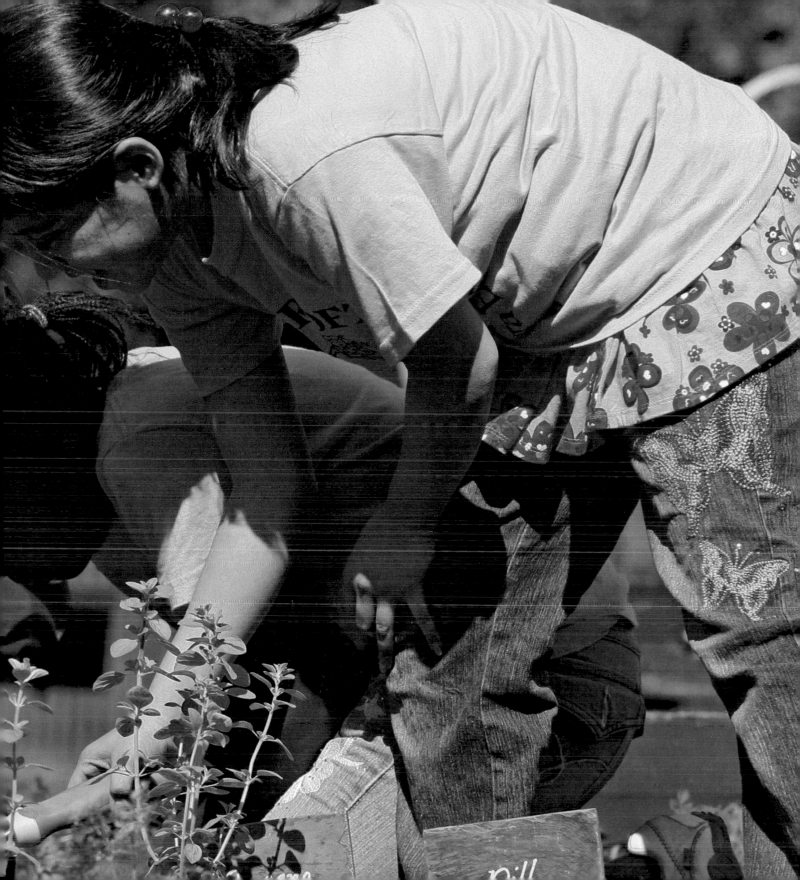

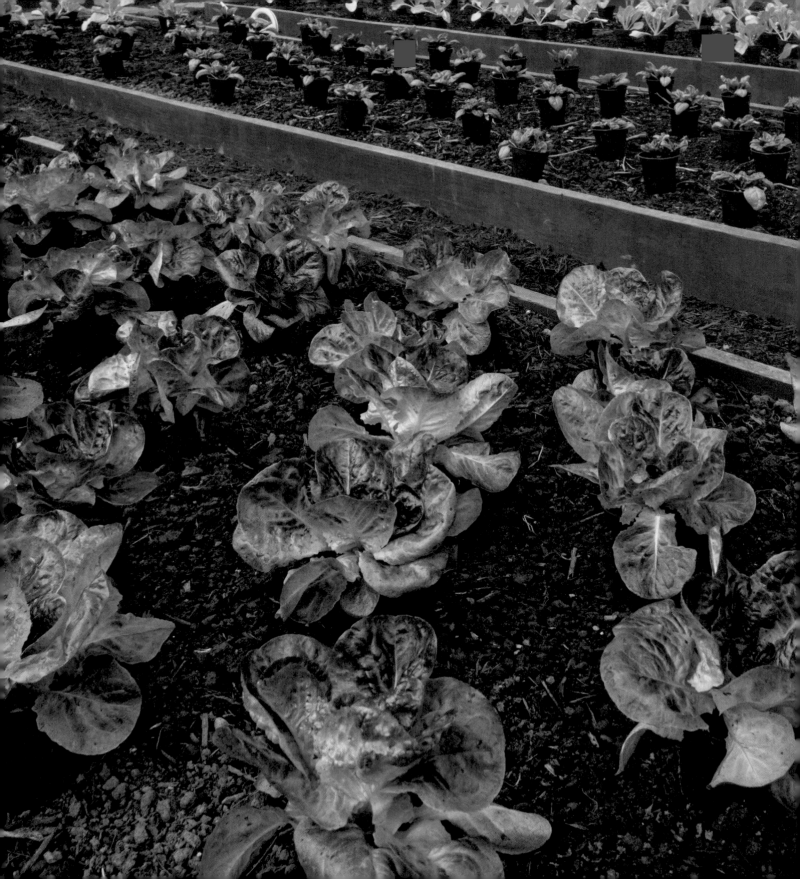

Spring: A Season of Hope and New Beginnings

For me, spring has always been a season of hope and a time for new beginnings. Such was the case with our White House Kitchen Garden, which marked the beginning of a learning process for all who planted and tended it. Our garden also helped us begin a national conversation about the food we eat and the impact it has on our children's health. Ultimately, the White House Kitchen Garden is an expression of my hopes for them: Just as each seed we plant has the potential to become something extraordinary, so does every child.

I first had the idea to plant a vegetable garden at the White House in my kitchen back in Chicago. It was early in the presidential primary season—the Iowa caucuses hadn't even happened yet. In recent years, I had been thinking a great deal about how the food my family ate affected our health. And as I was putting dinner on the table that night, I thought to myself that if something amazing happened, if my husband—then very much the underdog in the race—actually won, then as first lady I might want to focus on this issue more broadly. That night, it occurred to me that planting a garden at the White House—a garden where children could learn about growing and preparing fresh, nutritious food—could be one small way to get started. As the primary season, and then the general election season, wore on, I kept the idea of that garden in the back of my mind. Soon after my husband was elected, I began to think about how to make it a reality.

Bo by the Jefferson beds.

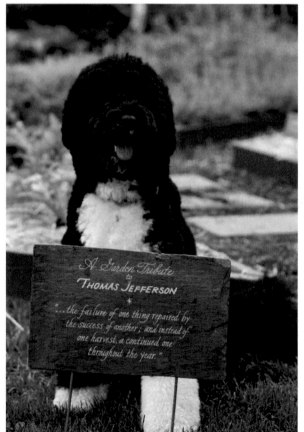

A Brief History of Gardens at the White House

Our second president, John Adams, was the first to live in the newly built White House, though only for four winter months. He had the ground plowed and fertilized for its first "kitchen garden" (such gardens supplied fresh produce to the kitchen and were often located near the kitchen door), though no one knows exactly where it was located. He lost his bid for reelection and departed the White House in March 1801; his garden was never harvested.

Fortunately, America's third president, Thomas Jefferson, was an avid gardener. When Jefferson arrived in Washington, the White House was not yet complete. Trees had been cut down for firewood, and their stumps were left behind. Briar bushes covered the road between the White House and the Capitol. But President Jefferson was undeterred.

He began by enclosing a small area around the White House with split-rail fences. He then lined the grounds with groves of trees and even started growing plants inside the

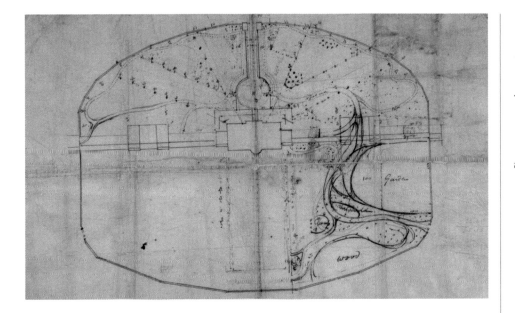

White House itself, arranging pots of geraniums and strawberries and fig and orange trees along three sunny window bays in his office.

Although Jefferson never planted a White House kitchen garden, he was constantly experimenting with new seeds and plants at Monticello, his home located just outside of Charlottesville, Virginia.

In 2010, my daughters and I had the pleasure of visiting Monticello, and we walked the grounds with Peter Hatch, the Director of Gardens and Grounds, who graciously provided seeds and seedling plants for our White House garden. We learned that President Jefferson grew more than 100 species of flowers and 330 varieties of vegetables and herbs, many of which are extinct today. He kept pages of notes on his garden, and his letters are filled with garden questions, thoughts, and updates.

Peter told us some wonderful stories about Jefferson. Apparently, at the age of eighty-three, the former president became obsessed with four-foot-long cucumbers. He had read about them in an old newspaper, and he

THE JEFFERSON BEDS

Two of our thirty-four beds are dedicated to Thomas Jefferson, and the plantings in these beds are grown from seeds collected from the gardens at Monticello. Jefferson never wrote his memoirs; instead he built them into his house and his grounds. His gardens became a showplace, an experimental laboratory where he cultivated the local and the exotic. Growing now in our beds are some of Jefferson's favorite vegetables, including Tennis-ball and Brown Dutch lettuces, Green Globe artichokes, and Marseilles figs.

Jefferson was a great collector of plant specimens and seeds, and he readily shared what he grew with his neighbors around Monticello. I like to think about those seeds traveling back to the White House more than two hundred years later to take up residence in this ground.

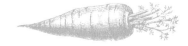

became determined to grow them in his own garden. It wasn't easy, but Jefferson was willing to endure repeated failures in the hopes of achieving just one success. His persistence is captured in the quote we chose to honor the Jefferson beds of our garden: ". . . the failure of one thing repaired by the success of another; and instead of one harvest, a continued one throughout the year." This has become the guiding principle for our Kitchen Garden.

Unfortunately, much of Jefferson's work at the White House was lost when the British trampled the grounds and set fire to the house during the War of 1812. But by 1825, yet another gardener had moved in: President John Quincy Adams. As he traveled, Adams liked to gather interesting seeds and dig up small plants. He would carry them back in his coach and plant them at the White House. The next president, Andrew Jackson, planted trees of all shapes and sizes, and he began the tradition of planting hundreds of bulbs that bloomed in the spring.

Throughout the nineteenth and early twentieth centuries, the White House grounds continued to evolve. President Ulysses S. Grant added ornamental fountains, and First Lady Edith Roosevelt, President Theodore Roosevelt's wife, planted a colonial-style garden next to the residence. Two presidents later, First Lady Ellen Wilson replaced Edith's garden with the formal, rectangular rose garden that remains there today.

By the early 1930s, so many presidents had left their own marks that the White House grounds were a hodgepodge of styles and designs. That all changed in 1935, when President Franklin Roosevelt asked Frederick Law Olmsted Jr., a landscape artist, to design a plan for the grounds. Olmsted created the South Lawn, which looked more like a park, with groups of trees and rolling lawns. He kept the Rose Garden

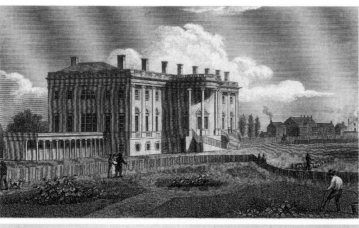

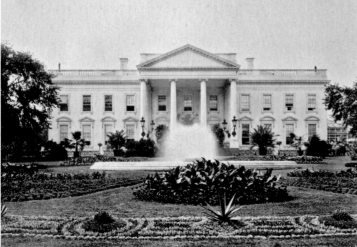

WHITE HOUSE GARDENS IN THE 1800S

The 1800s were a time of great change on the White House grounds.
Top, an engraving depicting one of the earliest images of the home. Above,
a photograph showing the front lawn at the height of its Victorian splendor.

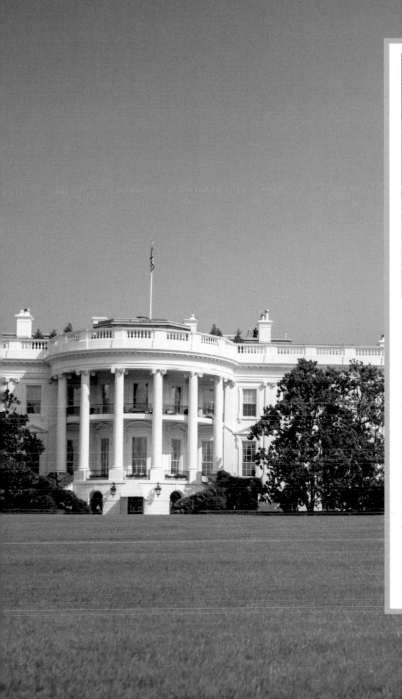

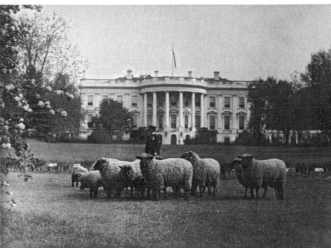

SHEEP GRAZING ON THE SOUTH LAWN

During the 1850s, the grounds were sometimes open
to the public, and well-dressed Washingtonians rode
their horses along the South Lawn's paths and walked
around its green spaces. By the 1870s, the Easter Egg
Roll and spring garden parties became the rage, and in
1911, several thousand people attended a garden party
hosted by First Lady Helen Taft in honor of her twenty-
fifth wedding anniversary. In 1973 First Lady Patricia
Nixon opened the White House grounds to the public for
a weekend of spring garden tours; her older daughter,
Tricia, had gotten married in the Rose Garden two years
earlier. And while there are some old photographs of
sheep on the South Lawn, keeping livestock there wasn't
common.

and a matching flower garden on the east side, but he took out all the other flowers, except for those around the fountains. Since Olmsted's plan was adopted, the White House grounds have remained largely unchanged.

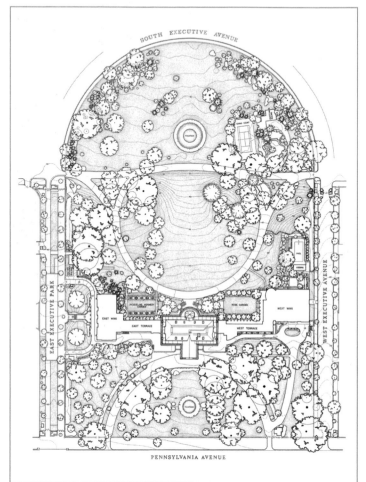

GROUNDS TRANSFORMED

Frederick Law Olmsted's plan for the White House grounds replaced masses of small flower beds and shrubs with a wide, sloping lawn and clusters of trees. His vision is preserved in the current landscaping, drawing above.

With the onset of World War II, much of America's canned food was sent to feed troops and civilians in Europe, so canned fruits and vegetables were less readily available. Consequently, many Americans began planting victory gardens in their backyards, which produced some 40 percent of America's food.

In an attempt to encourage these efforts, First Lady Eleanor Roosevelt decided to plant her own victory garden at the White House. Unfortunately, she ran into a series of obstacles. Soil tests on parts of the White House lawn came back showing poor soil quality, and the U.S. Department of Agriculture opposed the idea of a garden because they thought it might be seen as a challenge to American farmers, the nation's primary crop growers. But Mrs. Roosevelt prevailed, and a small garden patch was dug at the edge of a flower bed. The garden was tended by Diana Hopkins, the daughter of Harry Hopkins, one of President Roosevelt's top advisors. But this victory garden appears to have been more of a symbolic victory: No one knows what became of the food that was planted there.

Of course, there have been a few changes since the Roosevelt Administration. Trees have died or been knocked down by storms and have been replaced. President John F. Kennedy redid the Rose Garden following a design by the American horticulturist and gardener Rachel "Bunny" Lambert Mellon. The Rose Garden's plush lawn now looks like a thick grass carpet surrounded by roses and boxwood, and it can hold four hundred people at a public event. The East Garden (also known as the Jacqueline Kennedy Garden or the First Ladies' Garden), which is based on a traditional eighteenth-century

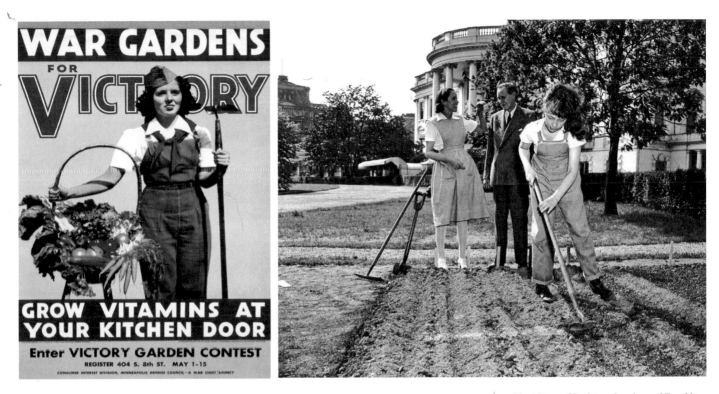

Here Diana Hopkins, daughter of Franklin Roosevelt's close advisor Harry Hopkins, tends the White House victory garden.

American garden, was completed under First Lady Lady Bird Johnson. Mrs. Johnson also added her own personal touch to the grounds, the Children's Garden. Created as a secluded place for children to play, it is tucked away toward the lower part of the South Lawn. The space we chose for our Kitchen Garden sits just below that garden.

Although President Jimmy Carter supported an herb garden for the chefs, and White House gardeners grew pots of tomatoes for President Bill and Mrs. Hillary Clinton and President George and Mrs. Laura Bush, not since Eleanor Roosevelt's victory garden during World War II had anyone grown food on the White House lawn.

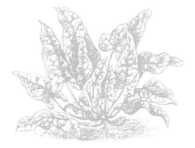

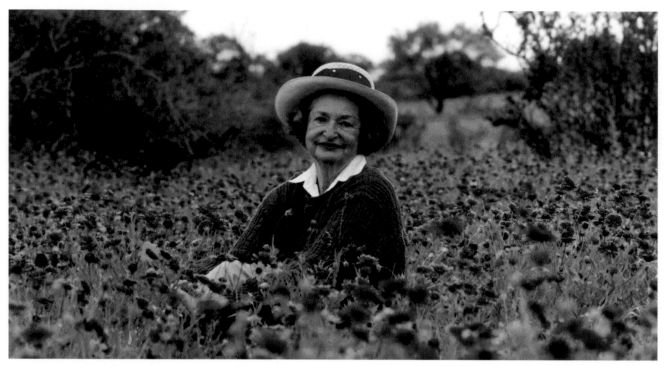

No first lady loved plants and gardening more than Lady Bird Johnson. She was particularly dedicated to preserving and protecting native plants across the country and in her home state of Texas, so that future generations could share in their beauty.

Once, during a Sunday drive in Texas, Mrs. Johnson spotted a farmer plowing up a field of wild pink evening primrose just as it was going to seed. Mrs. Johnson jumped out of the car and asked him to stop. For her conservation work, Mrs. Johnson received numerous awards, including the Presidential Medal of Freedom and the Con-gressional Gold Medal. She was affectionately described by former Secretary of the Interior Bruce Babbitt as "a 'shadow' Secretary of the Interior for much of her life." Many also hail her as a pioneer-ing environmentalist. In 1982, she established what is now the Lady Bird Johnson Wildflower Center in Austin, Texas.

At her ranch in Texas, Mrs. Johnson nurtured Texas bluebells and mesquite trees. She also grew colorful chrysanthemums that had first bloomed in the Alabama garden of her grandmother. When her plants grew too big, she would divide them up and give them away, allowing the blooms to thrive in other gardens. She loved the idea of linking generations of plants and people. Along with her flow-ers, Mrs. Johnson also raised peach trees, which produced peaches so ripe that, as she put it, "the juice would run down the back of your wrist as you ate it."

In her later years, Mrs. Johnson lived in a home in West Austin, Texas, that she had chosen because of the view and the flowering evergreen madrone tree in the front yard. Mysteriously, as Mrs. Johnson's health declined so did the tree's, and it died at about the same time that she passed away.

Planting Our White House Garden

The White House is actually considered a national park, so when I first moved to Washington, I wondered whether we'd even be allowed to plant a vegetable garden on the White House lawn, land that had been largely unchanged for decades. After talks with the National Park Service, I was thrilled to find out that the answer was yes, and in early 2009 we began to look for the perfect spot on the grounds. It needed to get enough sun and also be out of the main vista of the South Lawn but still be visible from outside the gate.

We sought advice from numerous farmers and gardeners, and came to rely on local farmer Jim Crawford, who would also help guide the design and planting of our garden. We eventually settled on a spot at the back edge of the South Lawn that could easily be seen from outside the White House gate. That was important to me because I wanted this to be the people's garden, just as the White House is the "people's house." I wanted people who were just walking by to be able to share in what we were doing and growing.

Next we had to test the soil to see if it would actually be able to nourish and sustain our crops. Because this was an urban site and we had no idea what had been put on, or in, the ground over the years, we all assumed that the soil on the South Lawn wouldn't be viable. But much to our surprise, the results of the soil tests were good. We wouldn't have to plant in raised beds; we could plant directly in the existing soil. All we needed was some good compost and a few additional nutrients to improve its quality.

We then had to decide on the shape of the garden. After much discussion, we came to a consensus on an L-shaped plot.

Finally, it was time to break ground. The White House gardeners had given us a hand by cutting down into the sod, but it still took a lot of effort to lift up the grass with our shovels and rakes. Fortunately, we had invited twenty-three fifth graders from Bancroft Elementary School in Washington, D.C., to help. Bancroft is a bilingual school with instruction in Span-

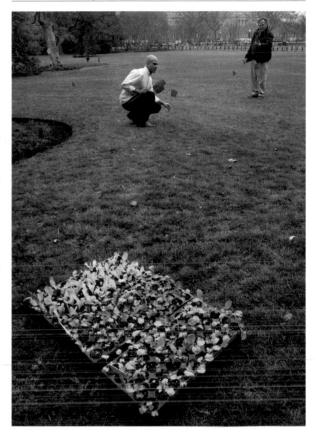

MAPPING OUT A GARDEN, MARCH 2009
Chef Sam Kass and White House Grounds Superintendent Dale Haney mark our future garden site with red flags.

ish and English, and it is home to students and teachers from more than forty different countries. Bancroft has its own garden, but even that didn't prepare the kids for how hard the work would be. Let's just say that we all got some good exercise that March afternoon. But breaking through the soil with our hoes and shovels was just the beginning. Next the National Park Service came through and pulled up what remained of the top layer of grass and tilled the beds with a rototiller until the ground was soft. Then we had to lay down additional sources of nutrients for the soil. Finally, it was time to sit back and wait for rain to water the ground and for the sun to warm it.

At last, the ground was ready for planting, and on April 9, 2009, I woke up feeling a little bit nervous. What if the seeds or seedlings were not set in correctly and we ended up with empty beds? What if we couldn't control the weeds? I worried about the weather, which I was discovering was no more reliable in Washington than it had been in Chicago. In the span of a day, it could turn from cold and dry to hot and humid. What if the plants just didn't grow? And what if, after all this effort, the food that did grow didn't taste good?

Fortunately, we never had to learn the answers to these questions. The garden took. As I had hoped, it also became a learning garden, and the garden team and I were among its first pupils.

SPRING PLANTING DAY
2009
There's magic in placing a new seedling in the ground and watching something you have planted begin to grow.

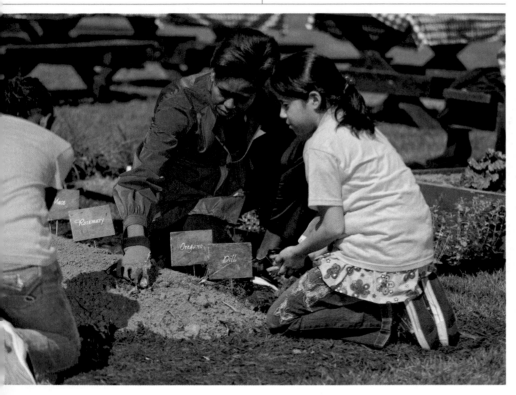

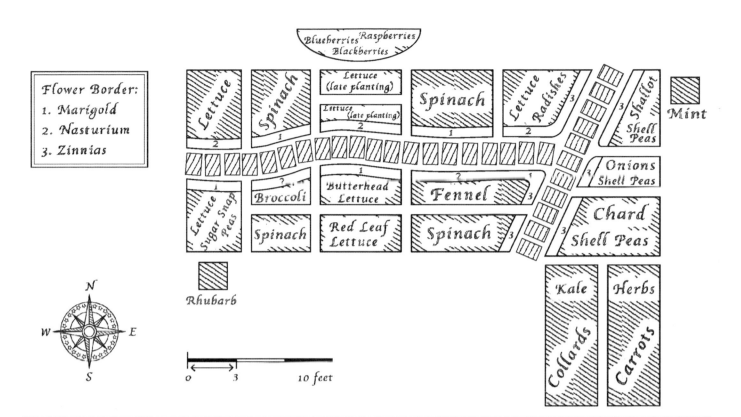

Flower Border:
1. Marigold
2. Nasturium
3. Zinnias

Blueberries Raspberries
Blackberries

Lettuce

Spinach

Lettuce
(late planting)

Lettuce
(late planting)

Spinach

Lettuce
Radishes

Shallot

Mint

Shell Peas

Onions
Shell Peas

Lettuce
Sugar Snap Peas

Broccoli

Butterhead
Lettuce

Fennel

Chard
Shell Peas

Spinach

Red Leaf
Lettuce

Spinach

Kale
Collards

Herbs
Carrots

Rhubarb

N
W E
S

0   3   10 feet

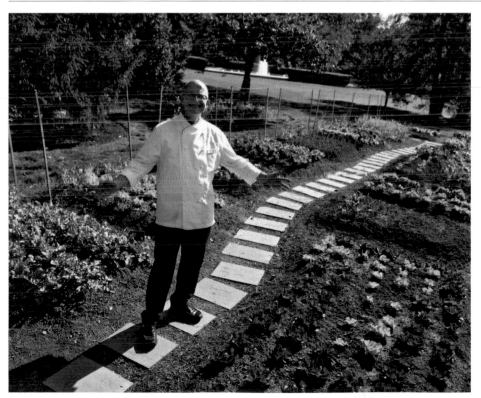

FIRST GARDEN PLAN

Our 2009 garden plan incorporated flowers
along with the vegetables and was about
four hundred feet smaller than the garden we
planted in 2012. Like most new gardeners,
our first year was a time for us to learn
from experience.

NEW BEGINNINGS

From the start, we wanted our garden to
be accessible so that school kids and White
House staff could wander among its rows.
Pastry Chef Bill Yosses admires our first
crop of lettuce.

MEET THE KITCHEN GARDEN TEAM

Our garden has flourished in part because of a wonderful collaboration between White House chefs and National Park Service gardeners. Together they select what will be grown in its beds, nurture its plants, and work with students and volunteers, sharing the lessons they've learned.

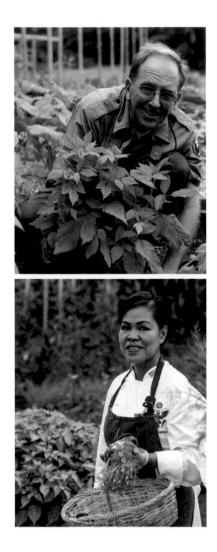

National Park Service Supervisory Horticulturist Jim Adams monitors every plant that goes into the ground at the White House. He keeps the planting records and oversees the changes in design. Many mornings, he is in the beds, clipping brown leaves, checking the moisture level of the soil, and making sure that the pea shoots really do climb up the fencing. Jim came to the garden with lots of experience, having spent nine years as the National Herb Garden Curator at the National Arboretum, where he was responsible for North America's largest designed herb garden, which includes annual, perennial, and woody herbal plants.

Executive Chef Cristeta Comerford came to the United States from the Philippines, a country where fresh food plays an important role in daily cooking, but this is her first experience with having a full garden. She has been the White House Executive Chef since 2005 and is the first woman and minority to hold that position. Cris works closely with Jim and Chef Sam Kass to select the crops and to incorporate our harvest into state dinners and meals for White House guests.

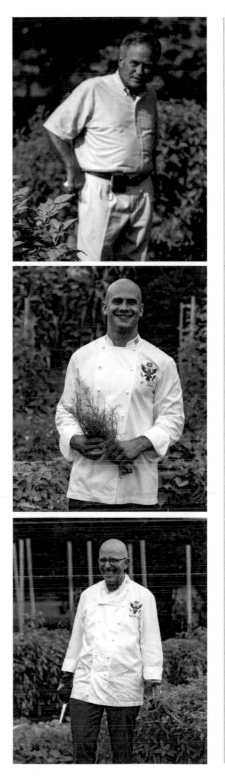

Superintendent of the White House Grounds Dale Haney hails from Pinehurst, North Carolina, and has been tending to the eighteen acres that make up the White House landscape since 1972. Dale oversees the day-to-day operations of the National Park Service, ensures that the grounds are in pristine condition, and selects the White House Christmas tree each year. And Dale doesn't just have a way with plants and trees, but with animals as well—he can often be seen surveying the grounds with Bo in close pursuit.

Chef Sam Kass helps select the crops, monitor the plants, and plan each crop season and harvest. Sam is also one of the chefs who wanders down in the late afternoon to harvest vegetables and herbs for the meals he cooks. In addition to his role as a chef, Sam is a senior advisor to my *Let's Move!* initiative, helping me work with businesses, schools, nonprofits, and others to solve the problem of childhood obesity.

Executive Pastry Chef Bill Yosses has worked at the White House since 2007. He first became fascinated by locally grown and sustainable food when he worked in leading New York City restaurants. While in New York, he helped develop Spoons Across America, a nonprofit organization dedicated to educating children, teachers, and families about the benefits of healthy eating. He finds that his work in the garden has taken him full circle, combining his passions for cooking, education, and public health.

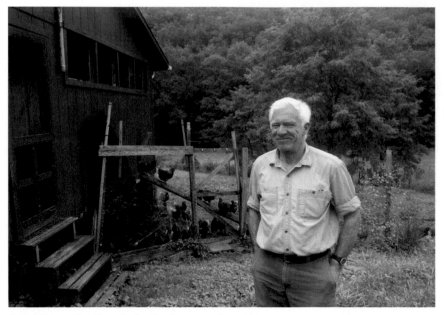

Local farmer Jim Crawford offered excellent advice on soil, plants, and design to help our Kitchen Garden take root.

Jim is an accidental farmer. He was a law student in the 1970s before he traded in his books for a tractor. Today, he and his wife, Moie, run New Morning Farm, a ninety-five-acre vegetable farm in south-central Pennsylvania, and Jim heads Tuscarora Organic Growers, one of the largest farm marketing cooperatives of local farmers in the nation.

"I started my first garden as a kid, beginning in the backyard, and then moving it to the front yard because the backyard didn't get enough sun. I was too lazy to keep it very well weeded. Thinking back on how the plot must have looked, my parents were very generous in letting me keep it there.

"If I was not a highly disciplined gardener, I was a very motivated one. I picked the food, ate it, and gave it away. But I never thought I'd be a farmer.

"When I was in my early twenties, I started law school and grew vegetables on the weekends. Pretty soon, I was farming full-time. Unlike a lot of farmers who grew up farming, I started with a really low level of expertise. I had to learn what crops like, when to plant, and what to watch out for. I read a lot of books, listened to a lot of other farmers, and slowly pieced it together. That learning experience is one reason I like to help other growers today.

"I still love farming, but it's a hard way to make a living, and the weather is always against you. In September 2011, our back creek flooded and destroyed one-third of our fields and our crop. As a farmer, you quickly learn patience—if it doesn't work one way, you have to wait another year to try something different. Farming is very challenging: You have to find a solution if something isn't growing properly, if the weeds are taking over, if there is some new disease. One of the hardest things now also is finding ways to sell a small or midsize farm to a new generation of farmers. In many cases, the land is so valuable that a young farmer can't afford to buy it and farm it.

"Yet even with all the challenges, farming offers something special, starting with independence. You are able to control your life and your business. And you build unique relationships. I sell cucumbers at our farmers' market in D.C., and one of our customers made pickles from them and gave us some jars.

"I used to worry that farming as a profession was dying off, but I see a renewal. We have more applicants than slots for our apprentice program. More young people want to go into farming. They've gotten the bug, just like me."

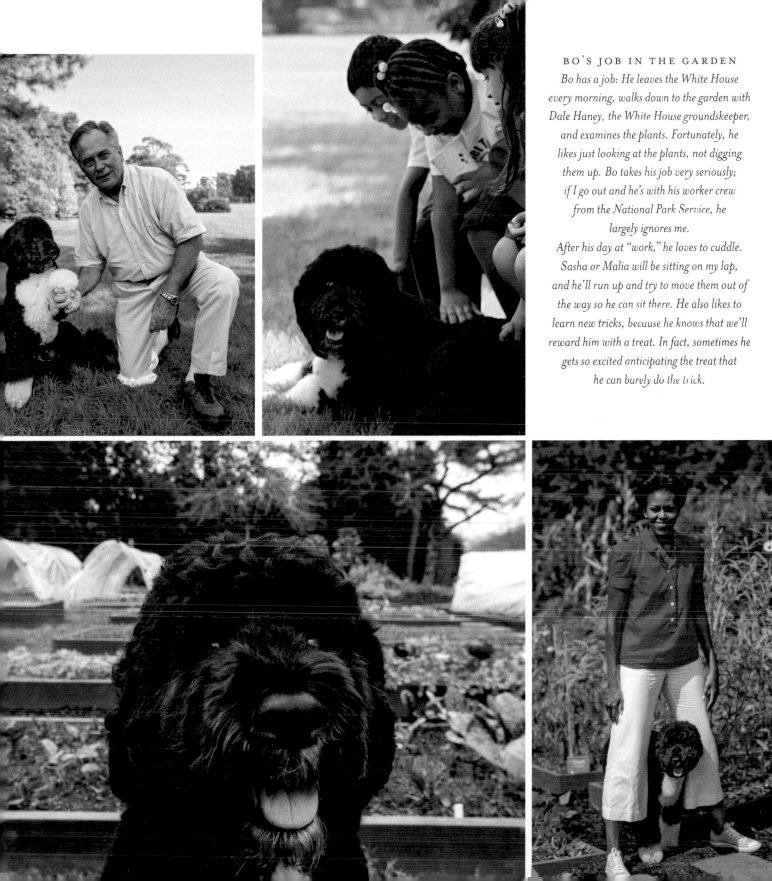

BO'S JOB IN THE GARDEN

Bo has a job: He leaves the White House every morning, walks down to the garden with Dale Haney, the White House groundskeeper, and examines the plants. Fortunately, he likes just looking at the plants, not digging them up. Bo takes his job very seriously; if I go out and he's with his worker crew from the National Park Service, he largely ignores me.

After his day at "work," he loves to cuddle. Sasha or Malia will be sitting on my lap, and he'll run up and try to move them out of the way so he can sit there. He also likes to learn new tricks, because he knows that we'll reward him with a treat. In fact, sometimes he gets so excited anticipating the treat that he can barely do the trick.

Beginner's Luck (and Misfortune): Lessons Learned in Our First Spring

When you plant a garden for the very first time, you wind up learning by trial and error, and we certainly had our fair share of the latter in the White House Kitchen Garden.

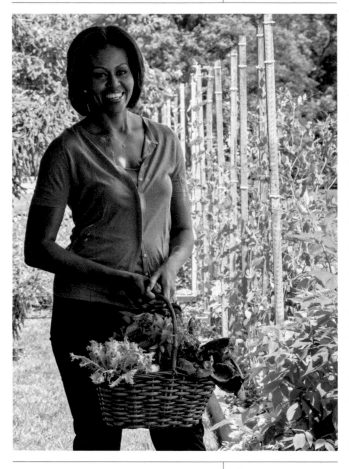

For example, we learned that the mounded beds—frameless, raised areas of soil—in our first garden were not such a good idea. For starters, they were too wide, so whenever anyone planted, weeded, or harvested, they were likely to step in the bed, compacting the fresh soil that the garden team had worked so hard to keep loose.

That first spring, we planted flowers along the edges of the garden to help with soil erosion and to make the beds beautiful. But we discovered that the flowers took up space needed for the rapidly growing vegetables. We also learned a hard lesson about the destructive power of rain—not the light, gentle rain that nourishes crops but the heavy, pelting thunderstorms that occur throughout the spring and early summer in and around Washington, D.C. The rain would fall in blinding sheets and wash away the mulch and topsoil onto the stones and into the grass paths. Once the skies had cleared, the top layers of the beds had to be carefully replaced, again and again.

There were also a few mishaps once the garden started growing. We grew beautiful, perfectly round cantaloupes that had absolutely no taste. We learned that our two blackberry bushes were taking up too much space for too few pieces of fruit. They never seemed to play nicely with the raspberry bushes beside them, always crowding and overshadowing them. We also had trouble with our blueberry bushes. We discovered that even with lots of netting, the birds still managed to eat almost every piece of fruit.

We've had our share of pests as well. While fences can keep out four-legged garden eaters, like rabbits and foxes, they can't keep out bugs. We've had infestations of cutworms (caterpillars that eat the stems of young plants) and also a bad invasion of cucumber beetles.

Over time, however, we came up with some pretty creative solutions to the problems we faced. We started enclosing new plants in bottomless paper cups to keep out the cutworms. During the spring and summer, the garden team now spreads a thin layer of straw on the beds to help control weeds and keep the soil moist when we hit a dry spell. The straw also protects the soil from heavy rains.

Over the years, we've rotated our crops, and we've also expanded our garden to make room for additional plants. We spent about $200 for soil, seeds, seedlings, and amendments (compost, lime, and other materials to improve the soil) for that first garden, and it wound up being 1,100 square feet in size and producing 740 pounds of produce by late October. Come spring 2010, we decided to add new beds, expanding to 1,500 square feet of planting space, including two more planting boxes for crops like rhubarb and sweet potatoes. We also trimmed some of the surrounding trees that were blocking the sun, and we worked out a better system for the water runoff, since the garden sits on the downward slope of the South Lawn. Finally, we traded in small raised hills of soil for wooden boxes (made of untreated wood, as pressure-treated lumber contains chemicals

OUR 2011 GARDEN
By 2011, everything about our garden had grown. We opened up more space and installed raised beds to protect the soil and make it easier to care for our crops.

WHY WE USE STRAW
In addition to helping control weeds, straw provides low-growing crops like melons, cucumbers, and squash with a protective layer on which to rest. This can help thwart rot. Both straw and other types of mulch also keep soil from splashing back on plants when they are watered, helping prevent some fungal diseases.

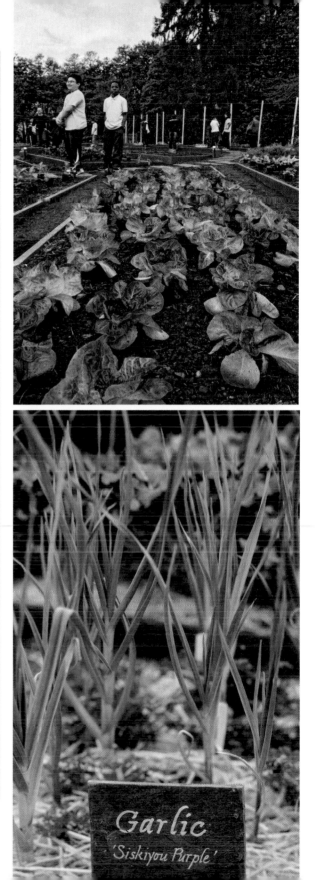

Garlic
'Siskiyou Purple'

that can leach into the soil), creating thirty-four separate beds, angled, shaped, and spaced just right for a child, or even an adult, to fit between. Through the seasons, the soil became richer as the boxed beds made it possible to retain more of the nutrient-rich compost. There were also plenty of earthworms in the ground to break up the soil and allow water to reach the roots of the plants, making it easier for them to grow.

WHY SPRING IS MY FAVORITE SEASON

The garden is prettiest—and most bountiful—in the very early part of summer. If you don't get down there every couple of days, it's like a child you haven't seen for a few months who has suddenly had a huge growth spurt. It sprouts up like a rain forest, and the vegetables are finally recognizable as food, not just a bunch of plants and flowers.

But my own favorite season is still spring, especially those last weeks of May and the start of June, when it is a nearly perfect time to be outside. The days are long; everything is vibrant and blooming; and I can sit outside without a jacket and watch the kids play with Bo on the lush green lawn.

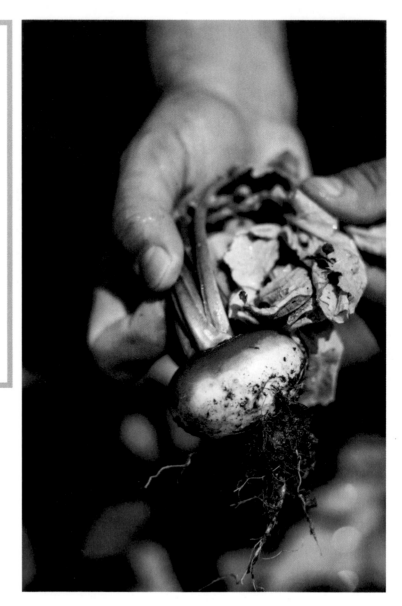

FRESH FROM THE EARTH
A Kitchen Garden turnip, just plucked from the ground.

MY SPRING-GREEN GARDEN GLOVES

During a visit to Toledo, Ohio, in June 2011, my husband decided to surprise me. He didn't hop off Marine One carrying a bouquet of flowers; instead, the package in his hand was a pair of bright green gardening gloves, purchased at Fred's Pro Hardware. The gloves have been my go-to pair in the garden ever since. And I like the green, because no matter what season it is, it makes me think of a perfect spring day.

The Very First White House Beehive

Bees are vital to gardens around the world—much of the food we eat is courtesy of a bee that has pollinated a plant so that it can bear fruit. But that first spring, it took some convincing for me to say yes to a beehive on the South Lawn of the White House. As someone who has always lived in a city, I had a vision of clouds of swarming bees around our family. But as I learned more, I found out that most honeybees actually don't like to sting people. Honeybees die after they sting, and as Sam Kass likes to ask the kids who come to visit the White House Kitchen Garden, if you knew that if you punched someone just one time, you would die, would you do it? The kids always yell, "No!" And that's the case for the bees as well. If you don't go messing with them, they won't go messing with you.

But there was one more person who still had to be persuaded: the President. When we told him about our plans for the hive, he was less than enthusiastic. The best spot for a hive was not too far from the basketball court where he likes to play, and he was worried about the girls, and even Bo, getting stung. But eventually, he came around to the idea, and we began the process of creating a home for our bees. We placed their hive high off

THE BEEHIVE

Beehives are replicas of the bees' traditional home, a hollow opening in a tree. Just as in a tree (below, left), our bees locate the wax combs for their brood in the lower part of the hive. The upper part is where they store the excess honey, in boxes called honey supers.

These boxes (below, center) got their names because they are "superimposed," or stacked one on top of another. During peak honey producing times in the late spring and early summer, we can have six supers stacked on our hive.

The bees cluster to fill the honeycomb cells (below, right). Each bee produces only $\frac{1}{12}$ tablespoon of honey in its lifetime. A summer bee's average life span is six weeks.

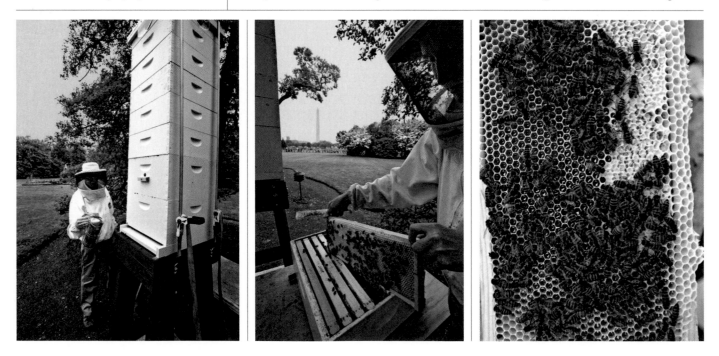

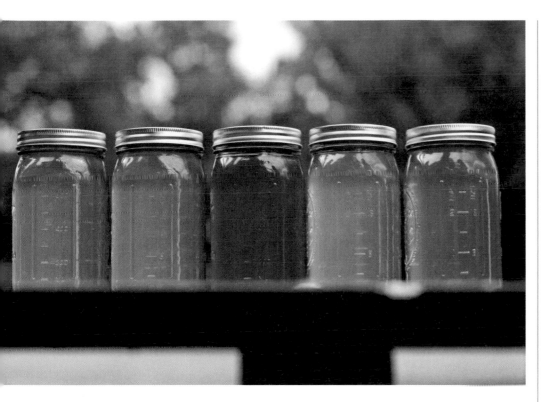

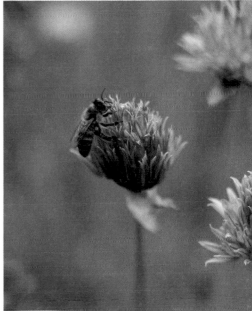

The jars of rich White House honey that we give, share, and enjoy begin with a honeybee gathering nectar from a flower.

the ground, to keep its entrance well above the kids who visit the garden and away from Bo, and it faces southeast, so the bees' flight path is in the opposite direction of the basketball court. We also made sure to strap it securely so that the winds from the presidential helicopter, Marine One, wouldn't tip it over during landings on the White House lawn.

At its peak in the summer, the hive is home to about seventy thousand bees. We harvested nearly 140 pounds of honey in our first year, 183 pounds in our second, and in 2011, the hive produced 225 pounds of honey. Some of the honey is used in the White House kitchen to sweeten everything from tea to salad dressings to desserts. We also donate some honey to Miriam's Kitchen, a nonprofit organization serving homeless individuals in the D.C. area (to which we also donate about one-third of our garden produce), and the remainder is bottled and given as gifts, often to visiting dignitaries and heads of state.

THE BEE SEASON
Charlie Brandts

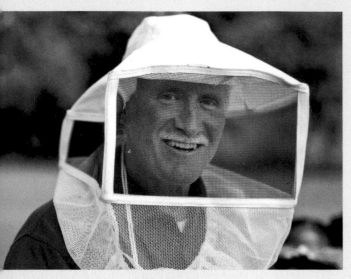

I've been a White House carpenter for almost thirty years, and I started raising bees at home about six years ago. I wanted something that would help keep me active, and I wanted to eat more healthily. One part of that was replacing table sugar with honey, and I found that there is no honey like the honey you raise on your own. What started small at my house has now grown to several dozen active hives. At the White House, one bee colony is enough to supply all our needs.

TALKING HONEY

"Bees and honey are two of nature's miracles. A honeybee can carry nearly its entire body weight in nectar. To fill its honey stomach—which it uses like a nectar backpack—just once, a bee visits between fifty and one hundred flowers. Back at the hive, worker bees 'chew' the nectar for about a half hour, then deposit it throughout the honeycomb."
—Charlie Brandts

I brought the bees to the White House from one of my hives and assembled their home myself. The big boxes on the bottom of the hive are the brood chambers, where the new bees are raised. The green boxes on the top are the honey supers, where the colony produces its surplus honey. We harvest honey from the hive from late June through late August, and I do it the traditional way: I create a little smoke to disrupt the bees' flight path and then lift out the frames and the cells. We spin the frames in the White House kitchen, which separates the honey.

Inside the hive, all the worker bees are females, and they're in charge of feeding the queen and the larvae. They also guard the entrance to the hive, collect nectar, and produce the wax comb, which makes our honeycomb. The male bees, the drones, have one purpose: to mate with the queen bee—and it's a pretty thankless job. Any drone that mates with the queen dies afterward. Any drone that doesn't mate with the queen lives but is cast out of the hive in October.

A honeybee's wings beat more than eleven thousand times per minute, which is what gives them their distinctive buzz. The bees can survive in the hive even in the middle of January because they vibrate their wing muscles to keep warm (they fan their wings to cool off in the summer). I love sharing facts like these with the children who visit the garden and the hive.

Kids come on tours, but they also come to help Mrs. Obama harvest and plant the garden. My most exciting day in the garden was during one of those plantings. In April 2009, we had seedlings spread all around the garden and were waiting for the schoolchildren who would help Mrs. Obama plant the garden for the very first time. On each box of seedlings, there must have been at least a dozen bees who settled down to drink off the freshly watered plants. The bees didn't think they were disturbing anyone, but the staff was feeling a little panicky. The kids were coming, and Mrs. Obama would be there soon. They called me for help, and I immediately called the editor of *Bee Culture* magazine for advice. He suggested we block the entrance of the hive so bees inside wouldn't leave, and then pull the top box on the hive forward to entice the bees outside of the hive to come home. It worked! We managed to get all the bees to return to the hive. Bee-free, the planting was a huge success.

Later that day, I was down by the hive and looked up to see President Obama walking down to the garden with Secretary of State Hillary Clinton. I tried to hide behind the hive, but the President saw me and called out, "Are those bees going to swarm when I play basketball?" I told him, "Sir, these bees are more interested in nectar than in politics."

A BEE-UTIFUL APPLE TREE

For twenty-five years, a lone apple tree stood tucked away in the Children's Garden at the back edge of the South Lawn—but it had never produced a single apple. Shortly after we installed our hive, however, our bees took it upon themselves to pollinate this tree. It soon began to bloom, producing baskets of apples the size of small grapefruits—apples that were crisp and juicy and really, really good. Then that winter we had "Snow-maggedon," two powerful back-to-back snowstorms that dumped more than two feet of heavy, wet snow on most of Washington. Plants and shrubs were crushed, branches broke, and trees fell. When the snow stopped, the National Park Service realized that one of the casualties was our apple tree. But thanks to the bees, our tree had its one glorious season, and we eventually decided to plant another apple tree on the same spot. It will be several years before we have any apples again, but I'm sure they will be well worth the wait.

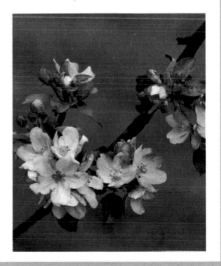

THE GREAT NORTHWEST GATE BEE CAPER

Bees outside of the beehive area of the South Lawn are a rare sight. But it did happen once, and we were glad to have Charlie and his expertise.

"I got a call that there was a swarm of bees at the Northwest Gate, the White House gate for the press and many presidential office appointments. I raced to gather my beekeeping equipment. When I arrived, I found Secret Service officers huddled in the guard booth and a group of reporters nearby. I quickly spotted the swarm of bees around a bush. Most people don't realize that honeybees aren't aggressive but defensive, and if you get the bees' wings wet, they can't fly until they dry off. I put on my suit and got out a water spray bottle and a big cardboard box. I then started spraying the bees and transferring them to the box. I knew that if I could get the queen in the box, the rest of the bees would follow. Fortunately, I was able to do so, and within ten minutes, every bee had joined her. I took the box home to my house and started a new colony. Several generations of bees have actually grown from that very queen."

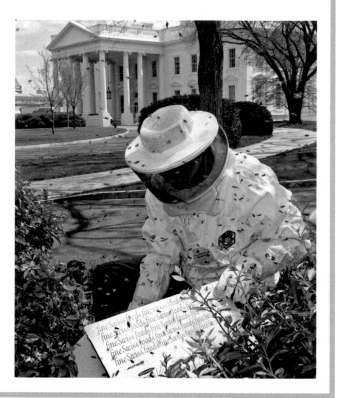

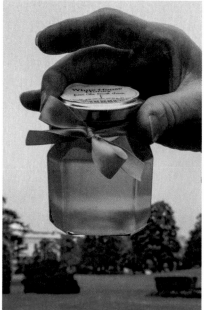

CENTRIFUGING HONEY

The honeycomb is a marvel of engineering: Each cell is only $^2/_{1000}$ of an inch thick, but it can support twenty-five times its own weight. A single frame filled with honey can weigh up to five pounds. Many people eat the honeycomb, considering it a delicacy.

🐝 We remove the frames and scrape off the wax coating to reveal the honey beneath.

🐝 Once the wax is removed, the frames that contain the cells are placed at equal distances inside a centrifuge to extract the honey. Just like making ice cream in an old-fashioned ice cream freezer, we crank the handle.

🐝 The spinning centrifuge releases the honey from the cells, and the rich golden liquid comes pouring out. Our honey has a light clover and basswood flavor, with a hint of citrus.

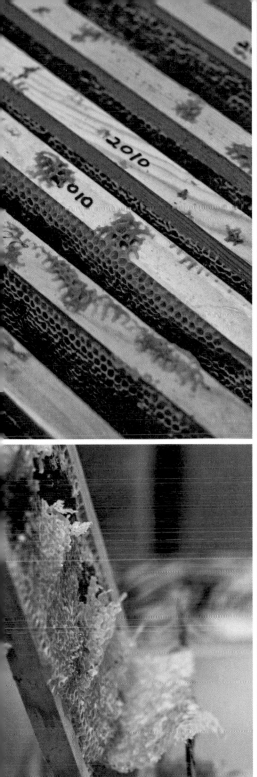
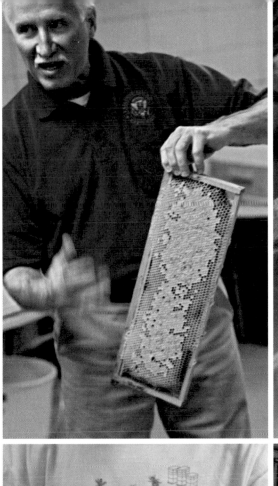
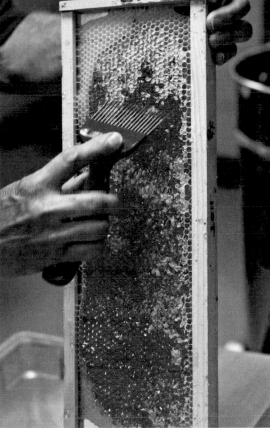
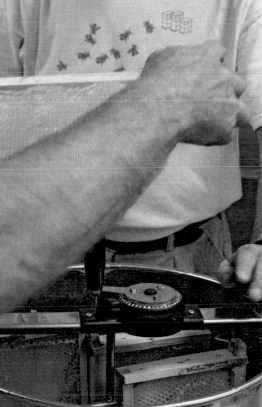
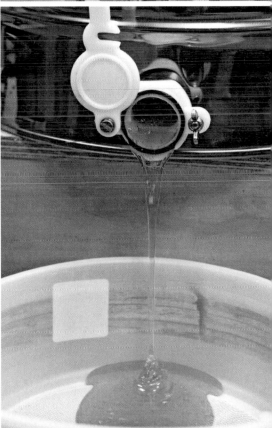

THE THREE SISTERS PLANTING, JUNE 2011:
CELEBRATING A NATIVE AMERICAN TRADITION

American Indians were our first gardeners, and we wanted them to have a special place in the White House Kitchen Garden. On June 3, 2011, American Indian and Alaska Native youth joined us to celebrate our nation's rich heritage with a traditional planting of the Three Sisters—corn, beans, and squash.

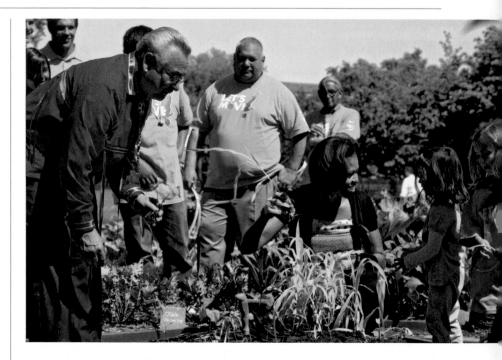

The Native Americans believed that corn, beans, and squash are like three inseparable sisters who can thrive only when raised together. Corn provides a natural pole for bean vines to climb, while the bean vines help shore up the corn stalks and leave behind nitrogen for the soil. Spreading squash shades the bed from weeds and keeps the soil moist. And all three plants create rich compost after the harvest. Corn, beans, and squash not only complement one another in the soil, they also complement one another nutritionally. Corn provides carbohydrates; beans, particularly dried beans, are rich in protein; and squash offers vitamins from the fruit and nutrient-rich oil from the seeds. Native Americans shared their Three Sisters planting system with early European settlers and taught them to recognize the signs that it is time to plant. On June 3, 2011, under a brilliant blue sky, we planted Cherokee White Eagle corn, Rattlesnake pole beans, and Seminole squash seeds, all donated by the National Museum of the American Indian. It turned out to be one of our most successful plantings in the garden.

PREPARING THE EARTH

We began the ceremony with a blessing by Jefferson Keel, Lieutenant Governor of the Chickasaw Nation and President of the National Congress of American Indians. Keel asked for "a special blessing on all things that God has created . . . and for the healing of Mother Earth and the seeds that have been planted so that they could continue to nurture us."

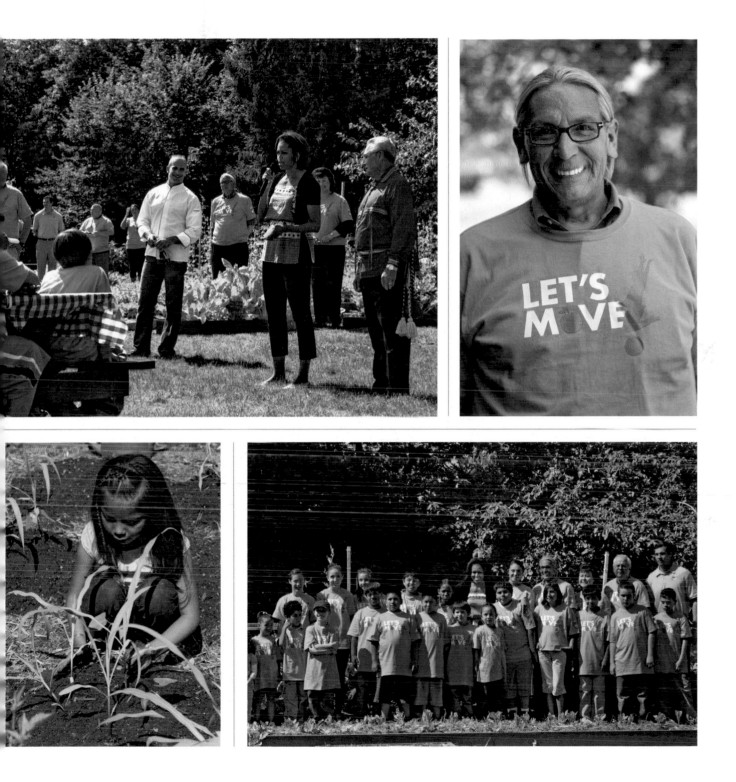

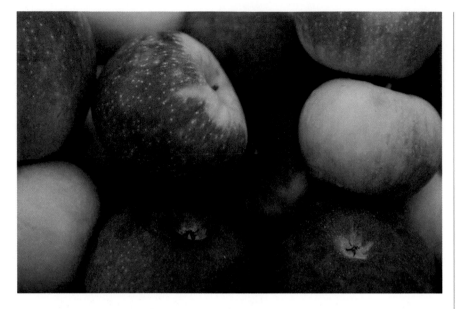

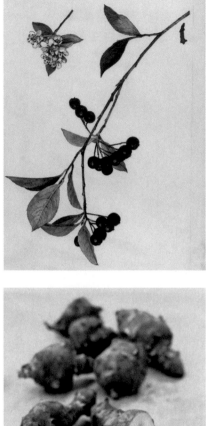

Before embarking on this garden journey, I hadn't realized that beyond blueberries, pecans, and a few varieties of grapes, the United States has few native plants that were ever part of our diet—and most of us wouldn't even recognize their names, like the pawpaw, the Jerusalem artichoke (also known as the sunchoke), and the chokecherry. Almost all of the vegetables and fruits we put on our tables today are "immigrants." Apples came from Asia; corn and beans came from South America; lettuces and cabbages came largely from Europe. Potatoes were actually first grown in the Andean mountains of South America, and initially many Europeans kept

IMMIGRANT PLANTS
Apples were a favorite of Thomas Jefferson, who liked them for eating and for cider. But apples aren't native to America. They were first grown in Asia.

them off their tables, but by the 1700s they had become a favorite crop. In America, they were made even more popular after Thomas Jefferson served them to guests at the White House. Tomatoes, a staple of Italian cuisine, came from Central America. But while people in the south of Europe liked tomatoes, northern Europeans thought they were unhealthy. In the United States, tomatoes became widely popular only after the Civil

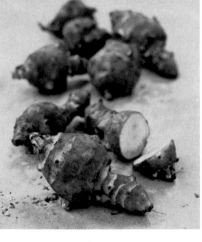

NATIVE GROWERS
Very few fruits and vegetables are native to North America, and many of them, like the chokecherry (top) and Jerusalem artichoke (above), are considered exotic today.

War. Now Americans eat more than twelve million tons of tomatoes each year.

By importing such a wide variety of fruits and vegetables, early American gardeners like Thomas Jefferson created, as Peter Hatch of Monticello put it, "a kind of Ellis Island" in their plots. Today, our White House Kitchen Garden continues that tradition and has become a melting pot of fruits and vegetables. In our first year, we planted cilantro, tomatillos, and jalapeño peppers, which are frequently used in Mexican and other Latin American recipes. We added collards and okra, staples of so much cooking in the American South. We also planted cabbage, a European staple, and we started growing ginger and bok choy, a tender Chinese cabbage.

The garden sparks international conversation as well. Whenever I have the privilege of traveling and meeting people around the world—from schoolchildren to kings, queens, and prime ministers—often one of the first questions they ask me is "How is the White House garden?"

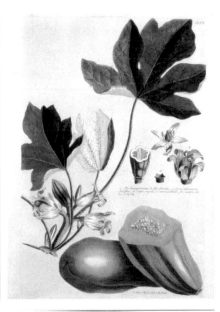

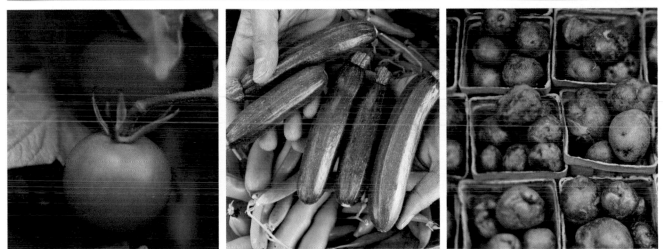

HERITAGE VEGETABLES

The flavors that are now so familiar to us are often the product of journeys between the new and old worlds. The pawpaw (top, right) is one of the few fruits native to the United States. Tomatoes and zucchini first grew in South America but were rebred when their seeds were carried back to Italy. Potatoes came from the Andes region near Peru, and it took hundreds of years for them to become a staple of northern European cooking.

The garden is not just a popular topic of conversation during our travels; it is also a wonderful source of gifts for people we have the privilege of meeting. Giving gifts to foreign dignitaries whom we're visiting abroad or who are visiting the United States is a time-honored tradition that helps us transcend cultural barriers and serves as a gesture of peace and friendship. A thoughtful and meaningful gift can instantly create a positive connection between leaders, expressing our appreciation of their culture and reflecting our pride in our own. Giving a gift from the White House Kitchen Garden is particularly special because it's personal (right from our backyard!) and involves something I love.

In 2010, to celebrate the sixty-fifth anniversary of the United Nations General Assembly, we gave visiting delegates a handwoven basket filled with gifts from the garden. Pickled vegetables, including tomatoes, cucumbers, carrots, peppers, okra, and herbs, were presented in glass jars. We also included tea made from chamomile flowers that were harvested from the garden for the first time that year.

In 2011, I traveled to the United Kingdom with my husband for an official visit. The United Kingdom's Prince Charles is an avid gardener, so when I was looking for just the right gift for him and his wife, I settled on seeds and plants from three very American gardens: the White House Kitchen Garden, Jefferson's garden at Monticello, and President George Washington's garden at his home Mount Vernon, in Virginia, as well as a jar of honey from the White House hive. Among the plants were a Brown Turkey fig tree from Monticello; boxwood from Mount Vernon; and Swiss chard, artichokes, and cauliflower from our own garden. The Prince subsequently planted our seeds and plants and even sent us photographs to show us how these transatlantic transplants were doing at his Duchy Home Farm.

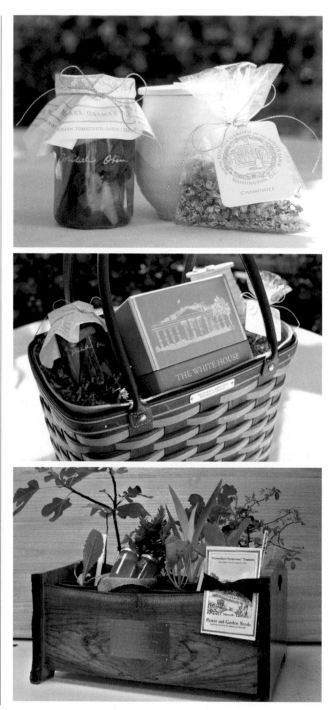

OUR MUSHROOMS

Each year in the garden, we like to experiment with a few
crops. In the spring of 2011, one of our chief experiments
was a set of mushroom logs. The White House chefs very
much wanted to have fresh mushrooms for the kitchen,
and so did I. We chose a shady spot under the pine trees
behind the garden, kept the logs well watered, and had
a bumper crop of oyster and shiitake mushrooms in the
late spring. Some mushroom varieties, like oyster, are a
good source of protein; in the right location and properly
cared for, a single mushroom log will usually produce
fruit in the spring and fall for anywhere from three to
five years.

Our Littlest Gardeners:
Planting the Seeds of Understanding and Connection for Our Children

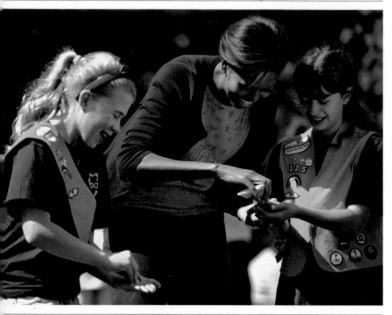

GETTING STARTED

Girl Scout Troop 60325 from Fairport, New York, came to the White House to help us with our Spring 2012 planting. These two girls planted some of the first seeds.

From the beginning, I knew I wanted children to play a major role in the creation and growth of our garden. I particularly wanted to include local kids who had never dreamed of visiting the White House despite living in the same city. The mom in me didn't know if they'd like getting their hands dirty or how they would respond upon encountering plump, wriggling earthworms in the soil. But kids are innately curious, and despite their reputation for being less than enthusiastic about vegetables, they are surprisingly willing to try new things.

We started with that group of students from Bancroft Elementary School, and we were determined to make our first planting day a great experience. We were highly organized: All the seedlings and seeds were pre-positioned by the garden beds, and the spots where they would be planted were already marked off in the ground. The kids were broken into small groups, and each group was paired with an adult: me, one of the chefs, or a special guest. Finally, after so many weeks and months of preparation, we got to planting.

On that day—and many days since—we discovered that our experience with children in the garden is about much more than just planting seeds and harvesting vegetables. Invariably, as we bend down and dig in the soil with the children, we start talking—about our lives and theirs. We've found that kids often want to sit by the adults and confide in us. They're eager to learn and be useful, and they thrive on knowing that grown-ups want their help and want to hear about what they're thinking and feeling.

In fact, equality is a key part of the message of planting day. We are all down in the dirt. Anyone present can help dig. There is no hierarchy, no boss, and no winner. It is almost impossible to mess up. We make it clear that gardening isn't about perfection. It's fine to drop a few extra seeds into

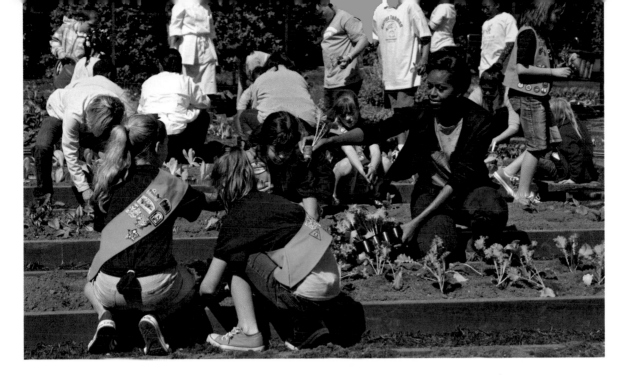

a freshly dug hole or even be short a few—as long as you cover them and water them well, a plant will probably sprout. I've always believed that kids learn the most when they're least afraid of making mistakes and they have the support they need to try, and fail, and try again. I want them to think: It's a plant, it's dirt, so don't be afraid; you can't ruin anything here, there isn't anything that can't be redone.

Each year, we've witnessed the impact of our approach on the lives of the kids who participate. As Cierra Beatty, a fifth grader at Bancroft, told me, "I like to garden because of the delicious food you grow. But I also like the garden because of how you can work together with other people on something fun." In the following months, Cierra and her classmates would return to see their plants grow and to harvest what they had put in that spring ground. They discovered that, as Carlos Aguilar, another fifth grader at Bancroft, put it, what they have grown tastes "good!" He added, "Planting these plants is special because they have been shared with us by the White House. Just as these plants were shared with us, we fifth graders shared in the planting of our own garden by inviting first and second graders to help us in the garden. We worked with them just as the White House cooks and gardeners worked with us. The sharing of good food has made us want to share good feelings."

After our first planting, in the late spring of 2009, I went to Bancroft Elementary to help the students plant their own garden and to listen to essays they had written about their day at the White House. One in particular, by a young man named David Martinez, brought tears to my eyes.

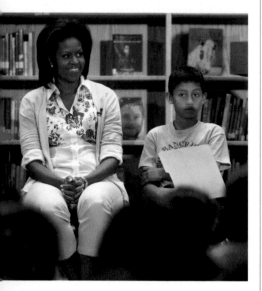

One of the things that I want to say about being at the White House was how gentle the feeling was. It felt surprisingly "natural" to be there. It was all about nature, and what is natural. We planted on a warm not hot day. The sun was out and there was a little breeze but no wind. The grass was beautiful and green. The people made us feel good. Mr. Sam, you remembered all our names, and shook our hands again. Mrs. Obama, you were working out there in the garden with us. Our White House partners for planting were helpful, but let us work too. They told us we did a good job.

I liked the way the staff person who helped me was very gentle with the worms we found. I watched how he gently pushed them back into their home, the soil. Respecting nature is also the theme that we heard from you, Mrs. Obama. You encouraged us to eat healthy foods, the red and green and yellow vegetables and fruits, so that we would take better care of ourselves. You explained that this was what the garden at the White House was for, and that those fresh foods were not just for your family but for all of the staff who worked at the White House. I liked the way everyone was included.

My teachers talk a lot about models for our assignments, and how we need to look at them and follow them when we do our own work. I think about the garden project as a model for being gentle: gentle with nature, gentle to your body, and gentle with each other.

—David Martinez

During each new season, as we plant our seeds and care for what we grow, I think of David's words.

Why Grow Your Own Garden?

Everyone has his or her own reason for starting a garden. Some people want to spend more time outside. Others are looking to be part of a larger community. But for many gardeners, the motivation may be as simple as wanting to eat fresh, delicious fruits and vegetables. As Carlos Aguilar, one of the Bancroft Elementary students, wrote in his essay about the White House Kitchen Garden, "The red in the tomato, the orange in the carrot, and the green in the lettuce leaf and broccoli stalk . . . we've tasted these colors fresh out of a garden, and they taste so much better."

There was a time when I had no idea that tomatoes didn't come in green plastic trays, covered by cellophane, and that they could be any color other than pale red. I could not even imagine the sweet, tangy taste of a tomato fresh off the vine. If I had eaten those types of tomatoes as a kid, I would have wanted them at every meal. And foods that travel a shorter distance from garden to plate don't just taste better—they often retain more nutrients, so they're better for our health as well.

We obviously can't grow everything that we put on our tables ourselves. But even the most humble garden—a pot in the window or a few staked plants in the backyard—can have an impact on our health and our enjoyment of the meals we serve our families.

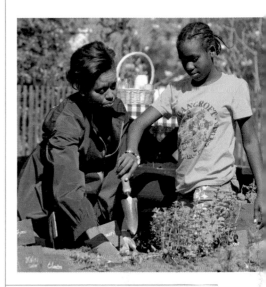

SPRING PLANTING DAY 2009
Planting herbs with the Bancroft fifth graders (above). We had a spirited discussion about gardening and healthy eating habits (below)

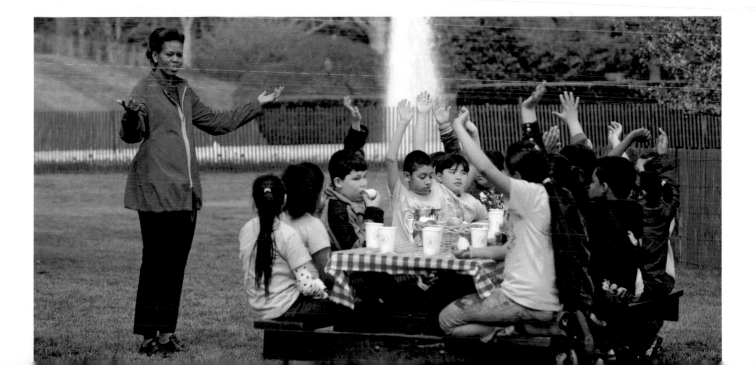

Building Your Own Garden:
Tips from Jim Adams, National Park Service Supervisory Horticulturist

IN CONTAINERS

Container gardens are a great alternative when you don't have time or space to plant an in-ground garden. If you have a sunny windowsill, patio, or balcony, you can grow your own bountiful harvest.

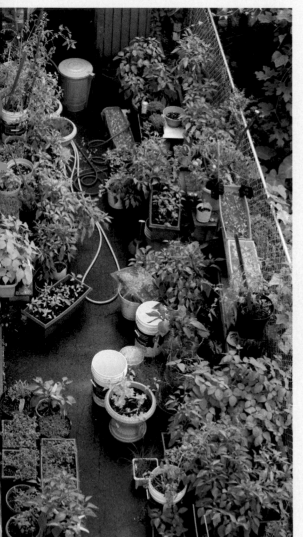

Sun equals success. You need six to eight hours of direct sun a day.

Potting matters. Soilless mix, which is made of lightweight planting material rich in organic components, is perfect for container growing. It retains just the right amount of water and can be found at most garden centers and nurseries.

Too hot to handle. Heat is often the biggest problem for container gardens. The soil in containers tends to dry out far more quickly than the soil in the ground. If the temperature rises above 90 degrees, container gardens may need to be watered twice a day.

Size matters. Make sure your containers are large enough and deep enough to hold your plants. Beans, cucumbers, and tomatoes require containers that are at least two feet in diameter or more. Peppers, greens, kale, and herbs can grow in smaller pots. Make sure that there is an opening and some stones or other substances in the bottom to allow for drainage so that water doesn't pool in the container.

Best bets. Tomatoes, cucumbers, lettuce, herbs, and peppers are all well suited to a container garden. Look for dwarf varieties or small sizes, like cherry tomatoes. Harvest salad greens lightly once a week to promote new growth. You can also double-plant in a container. For example, underneath your staked tomato vines, you can plant a small crop of herbs.

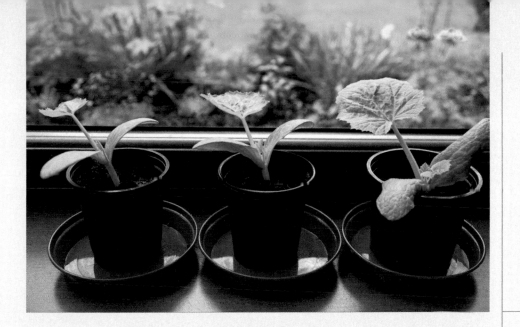

On Windowsills

No space for a backyard garden? No room for a container? You can still grow herbs and even small lettuces right on your windowsill. They'll just need light, water, and basic soil care. A two-foot-wide window box can hold four to six large herb plants or a small grouping of salad greens. Popular cooking herbs are a good choice, and many are easy to grow. Some window-box gardens even come preplanted, making this the fastest way to grow for the busiest lives.

In Your Backyard

Sun. Sun. Sun. The first step to planting a backyard garden is identifying how much sun your garden will get. Most gardens need six hours of full sun at a minimum. Even if you have a sunny garden, plant tall crops in the back of your rows or beds, where they won't block the light for small plants. Note that many plants, like tomatoes, prefer sun, but some, like lettuces, can thrive in a shadier environment.

How to find a sunny space. Here's a fun trick to find out whether you have a sunny or shady garden: Early in the morning, use twine and stakes, or a powder like lime or bonemeal (which is also good for your soil) to mark what part of the yard is shaded by a house or by trees or a fence. Go out again at noontime and see which, if any, areas are now covered by shade, and mark those areas. Go out one more time in the late afternoon to see which parts are now in the shade and which are getting sun. This will help you chart the path of the sun and show you which sections of your yard get the most sun and which get the least.

Before you plant, prepare. If you're planting in your backyard, it's important to test your soil to see if it has the nutrients necessary for a healthy garden. If you're gardening near a busy road or in a former parking lot or driveway, these tests will also tell you if the soil is safe. Once you've determined that your soil is viable, you will need to prepare it for planting. When we started our garden at the White House, we began by tilling the soil with a rototiller, which can often be rented from garden or home improvement stores. This process loosens clumps, mixes in nutrients, and creates a good base for what you will grow. In subsequent seasons, we've used shovels and digging forks, which are gentler on the ground.

Soil 101. Good soil makes a great garden. Soil is composed primarily of sand, clay, and silt. Soil that contains too much sand won't hold water and nutrients. Soil with too much clay is hard to work, often stays too damp after watering, and creates tough growing conditions for plants. A loamy mix, equal parts sand, clay, and silt, is the best environment for a vegetable garden. Don't forget mulch—a light one- or two-inch top layer of chopped leaves or a thin layer of straw discourages weeds and helps hold in moisture. As mulch breaks down, it also enriches the soil beneath. If you've invested the time to get your soil in great shape, you will spend less time keeping it up. Regularly working the soil—usually just once a week—with a trowel or a hoe will keep it loose and help keep out weeds. Regular weeding and watering is the key to garden health.

Water 101. Vegetables need at least one inch of water a week to thrive. That can come from rain, but when Mother Nature goes dry, gardeners have to pick up the slack. There are many different ways to water, though it's best to water plants in the morning so that the soil stays moist in the hot afternoon sun. Sprinklers and watering cans are good for newly sown seeds or just-

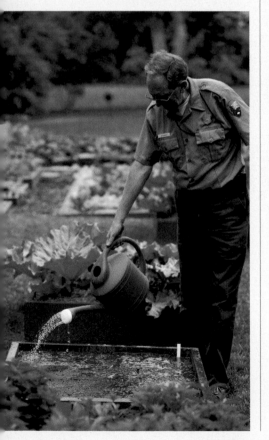

A GOOD SOAKING
Jim Adams, National Park Service Supervisory Horticulturist, gives new seeds a good soaking.

planted seedlings, which prefer gentle showers right on their freshly covered holes and new roots. After plants are established, try to water the plant at just above ground level. Getting too much water on the leaves and foliage can lead to fungal diseases. In the spring, the garden may need water only every three to four days, depending on your climate; and at the height of the summer, it may need water every day. You should periodically dig down into the soil to test its dampness.

What to grow. Grow what you like to eat. If you'll never eat kale, don't plant it. You can start with the basics: lettuce, tomatoes, cucumbers, and squash. Some of the easiest plants to grow are radishes, beets, tomatoes, and onions. Starting with plants from a nursery or seedlings grown from seeds sprouted in small pots on your windowsill may be easier for new gardeners. It is also important to select plant varieties that will thrive in your particular region of the country.

When to start. In Washington, D.C., it is possible to start planting cold-season crops in mid- to late March, but many regions of the country aren't ready for planting until May. In other areas in the South and West, you can plant almost all year long. Many gardeners use the U.S. Department of Agriculture's Plant Hardiness Zone Map as a guide. Most warm-weather planting needs to be done when there is no longer any danger of frost and the soil has warmed enough to allow seeds to germinate and roots to spread. But cold-season crops, like peas and lettuce, can be planted long before the last frost.

Here are the preferred planting and growing
temperatures for some garden staples:

55 to 75 degrees: garlic, leeks, onions, and shallots

60 to 65 degrees: beets, broccoli, cabbages, carrots,
cauliflower, kale, lettuce, peas, potatoes,
radishes, and spinach

65 to 75 degrees: beans, black-eyed peas, cucumbers,
melons, sweet corn, and squash

70 to 85 degrees: eggplant, sweet potatoes, sweet or
hot peppers, watermelons, okra, and tomatoes

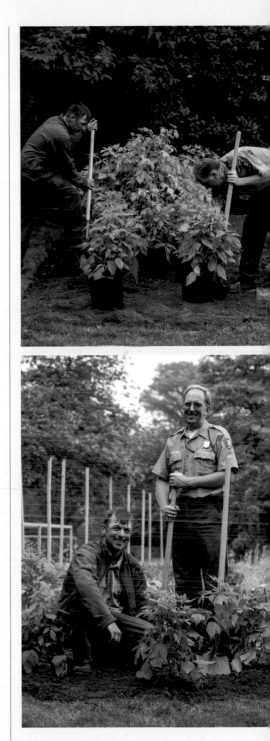

Jim Adams and James Pilkerton, Garden Supervisor, planting raspberries.

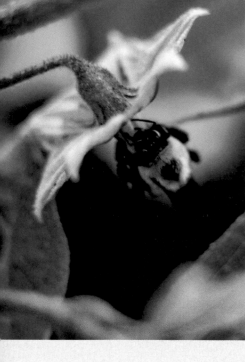

Wildlife. If you have a problem with rabbits, birds, or deer where you live, you may need to use chicken wire to protect plants. And if you grow tomatoes, gently tying them to stakes or frames helps to produce the best fruit and to keep it out of reach of hungry critters.

Weeds. Weeds deprive plants of water, nutrients, and sunlight. They can also harbor insects. Using a hoe or a fork to loosen and turn the soil between vegetable rows will separate weeds from their roots. Doing this early in the growing season allows vegetables to grow bigger, stronger, and taller than the weeds, which deprives the weeds of water and sunlight. Suffocate weeds by applying mulch or straw, which is our preferred method in the White House Kitchen Garden.

Diseases. Wet and cool conditions can make your garden a breeding ground for fungal diseases—and some fungi, like powdery mildew, can wipe out an entire crop. If you do find evidence of a fungal disease, tear out and destroy the affected plants so the disease doesn't spread to the rest of the garden, and do not use those plants in your compost.

Bugs. There are good bugs—bees, ladybugs, praying mantises, and lacewings are all good for the garden. But others, like mealy bugs, flea beetles, aphids, and white flies, can damage your plants. A strong blast of water from the hose can remove them from foliage, or you can pick them off by hand. Horticultural oils and soaps can also deter them—as can natural or nontoxic insecticides, depending on the insect—and can be found at a gardening store. Rotating your plants from season to season can also help prevent pest problems. Simply plant your new crop in a different space—one where you have not already grown vegetables from the same family—so it will be less susceptible to existing pests.

Great Soil for a Great Garden: Creating Your Own Compost

Compost puts organic matter and nutrients back into the ground, improves soil texture, and creates air spaces within the soil, breaking up hard clay and making the ground more hospitable. Compost also helps soil hold water and encourages a diverse ecosystem to grow in the ground. It is home to worms, healthy bacteria and fungi, and good insects.

Compost is made by combining browns and greens. Browns are carbon-rich materials, such as straw, wood chips, and leaves (and it helps to chop up or shred your browns as they go into the compost). Greens are nitrogen-rich materials, such as grass clippings and kitchen scraps. You can also use clippings from any garden plants you prune, as well as the stems and leaves from harvested plants or older plants that are finished producing for the garden. The key is to achieve a good ratio between browns and greens: about 25 parts browns to 75 parts greens. Compost can be made in a bin or a pile or even by digging a hole in the ground. Turning it periodically to mix the ingredients helps to break down the plant and other matter.

At the White House, we make our own compost. We use a system of three large wooden bins joined together. In one bin, we place organic matter, such as leaves, grass cuttings, and harvested plant remains from the garden, and then we add kitchen leftovers, like fruit and vegetable peels and eggshells (but never any meat, fat, or dairy products, which can attract rodents). We also add some finished compost to the mix, to introduce inoculants, the living organisms (bugs and bacteria, for example) that help break down the components of the compost. The materials then "cook" together in our bin, decaying and warming to a temperature as high as 140 degrees. We have a small fan to help speed the process, and we mix the compost around to help it break down. We then move it to a second bin, where it finishes decomposing. Finally, the compost is transferred to a third bin, where it rests and cools, becoming a perfect habitat for nutrients (and plenty of earthworms). It takes four to five months to transform our raw "ingredients" into a batch of compost ready to be spread over our soil and young plants.

The composting process reminds us that gardens are a great lesson in giving. The soil in the garden gives its nutrients to the plants it grows, so if

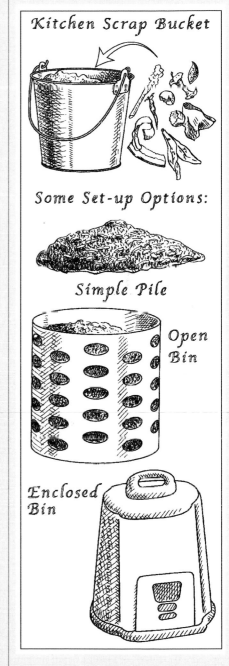

Kitchen Scrap Bucket

Some Set-up Options:

Simple Pile

Open Bin

Enclosed Bin

we want to grow the strongest, healthiest plants, we have to give everything we can to that soil. Composting represents a near-perfect circle of giving, taking our excess and turning it into something that can be reused to benefit the next generation of fruits and vegetables. It is a reminder that in gardening, as in life, we cannot just take—we need to give back as well.

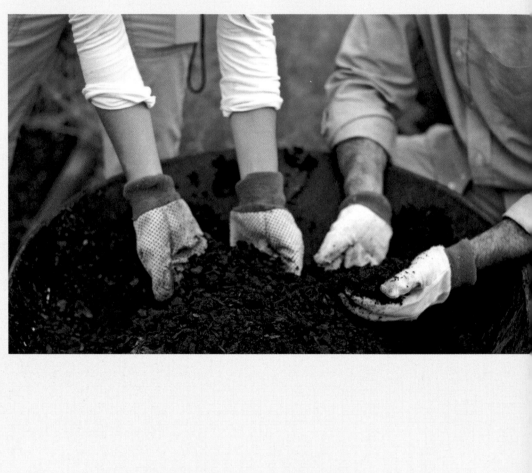

FRESH COMPOST

Volunteers prepare to spread fresh compost. Ours can take up to six months to finish "cooking" and decomposing into a rich addition for the soil.

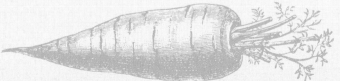

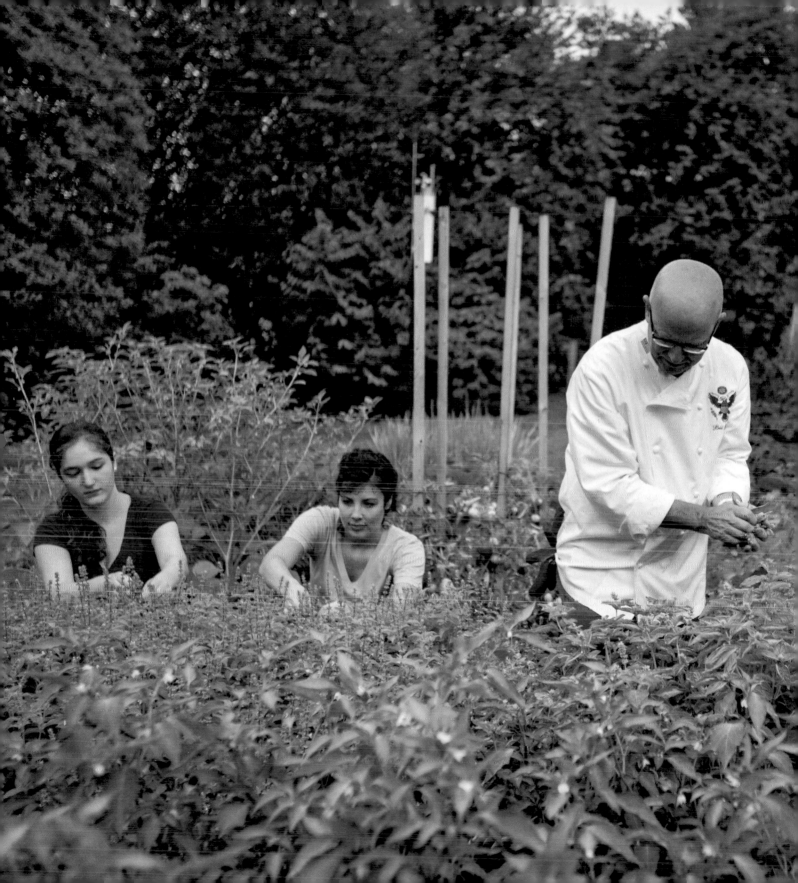

From the White House Kitchen Garden to the Table
Executive Chef Cris Comerford

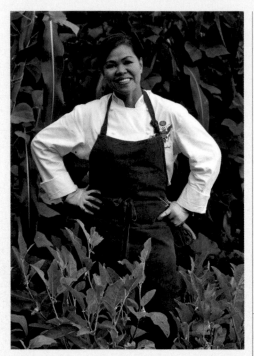

We plan our menus for events, large and small, by what is growing fresh in the garden. Our menus really revolve around nature, around what is out in the garden and ready to harvest. Since we planted the garden, I've noticed a change in what we cook. No longer are the meals we serve driven by the protein on the plate and garnished with a few baby carrots or other accent vegetables. Vegetables are now equal partners. And these aren't the vegetables from our childhoods, cooked until they've become mushy and turned a different color. When vegetables are fresh from the garden, you can simply sauté

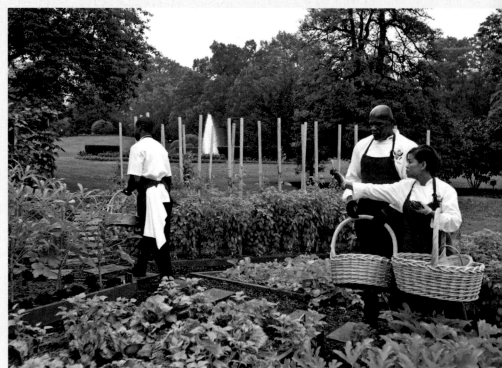

them or cook them lightly and add a few fresh herbs. And in many cases, complementary foods grow at the same time during the season. Tomatoes and eggplant, for example, share the same harvest period and taste delicious together.

After we harvest the vegetables, our first step is to weigh everything so we can keep track of how much is growing in the garden. If the harvest is largely greens, we wash them right away in deep sinks, with ice water, so they won't wilt. If it has been dry and dusty, we will need to wash the greens about three times to fully remove the dirt and sand. We then dry them very carefully in large salad spinners. Once they are completely dry, we store them in sealed plastic bags or sealed plastic tubs. If we have an official event or state dinner, we will use the crop there. And about one-third of what we harvest is donated to Miriam's Kitchen, an organization that provides meals and services for homeless individuals in the D.C. area.

Every crop receives its own special care. We leave tomatoes out on the counters to keep ripening. Sweet potatoes need to be cured—stored in a

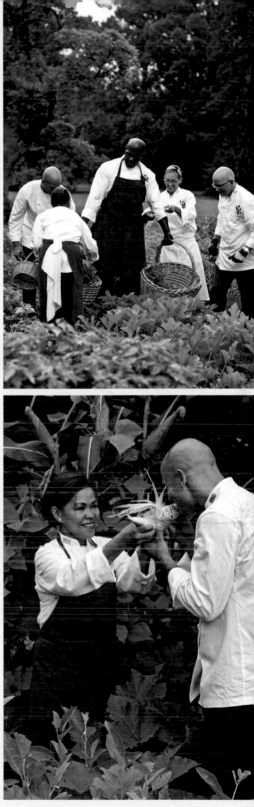

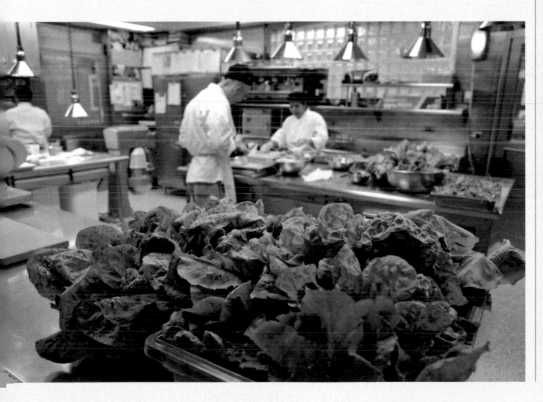

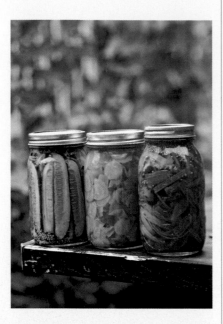

"Canning and preserving what grows in the garden allows us to serve flavors from the garden all year long. Quickly preparing a new harvest, whether it is lettuce from the soil or tomatoes just off the vine, is the key to maintaining its freshness."
—Chef Cris

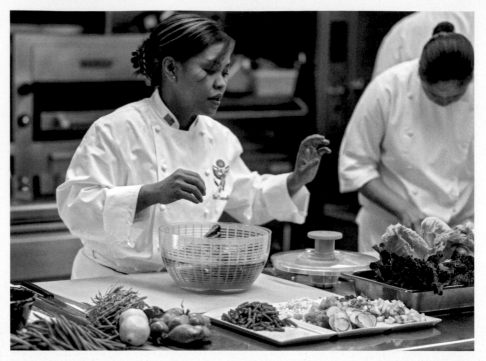

warm, humid room for several days—before they can be cooked. And in 2010, we started pickling some of our vegetables. When you see up close the hard work that goes into growing food from the ground, you feel a special obligation to care for it. Even as a chef, since we planted the garden, I've gained a new respect for the food that I cook.

My time with the garden has made a difference in my personal life as well. I want to be able to keep up with my ten-year-old daughter, who is a competitive gymnast, and I want to set an example for her with smart food choices. So today, at my home, I also try to serve a balanced diet with whole grains, low-fat proteins, and lots of vegetables. We save meals like hamburgers and fries for the weekend. I also dream of starting a garden in my own backyard, so I can put into practice for my family the lessons I have learned in our White House garden.

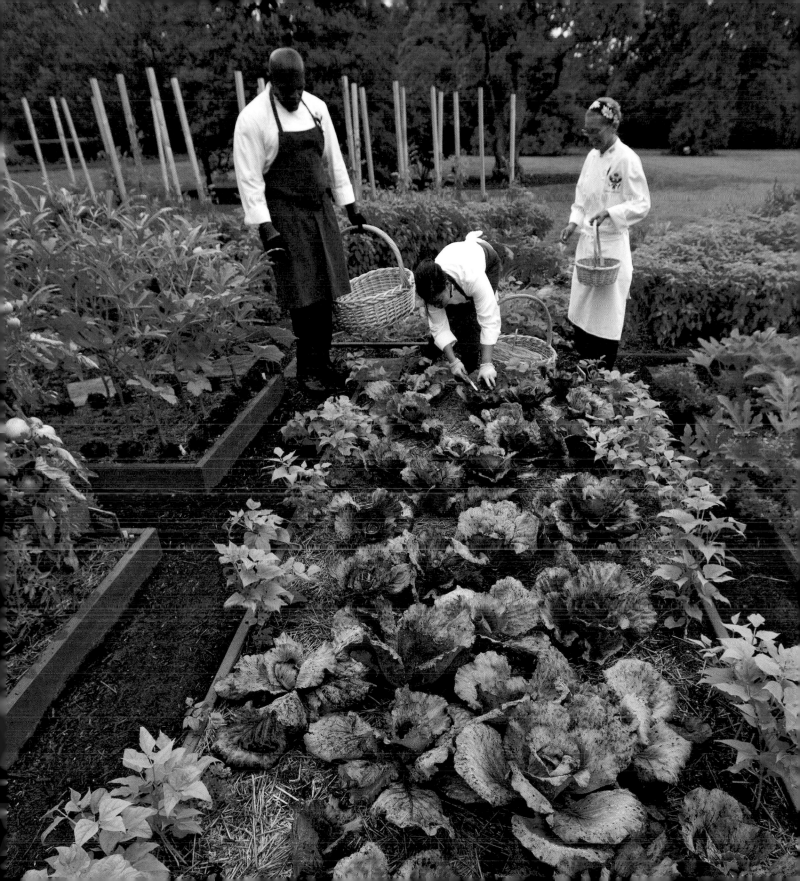

THE 2011
Spring Garden
PLAN

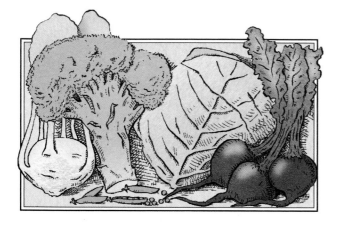

"Gardening isn't about perfection. It's fine to drop a few extra seeds into a freshly dug hole or even be short a few— as long as you cover them and water them well, a plant will probably sprout."

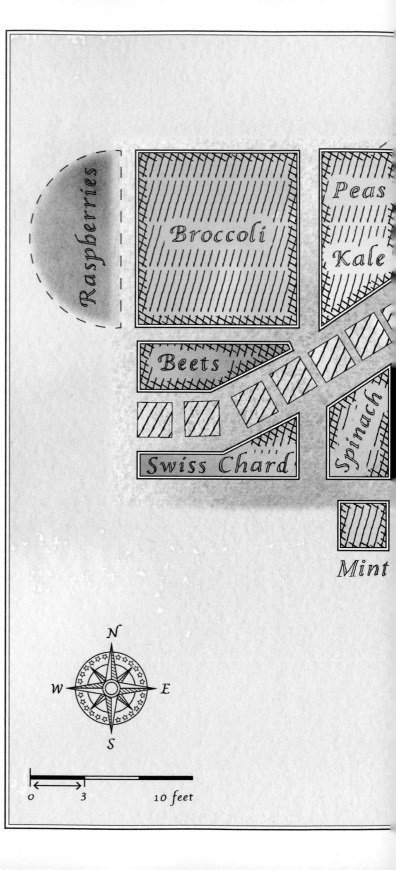

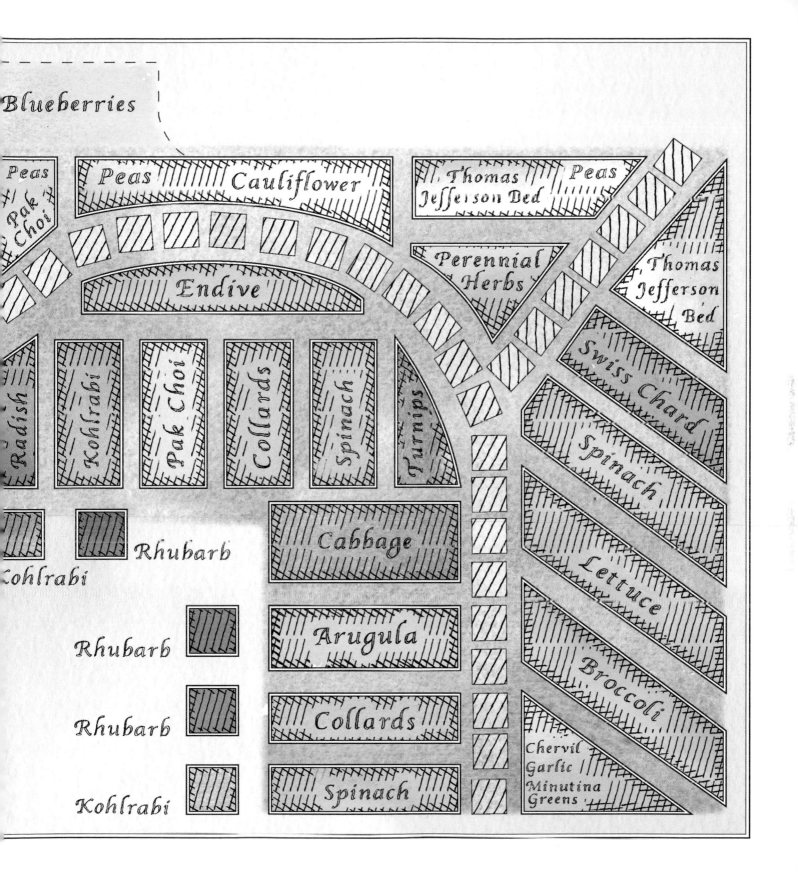

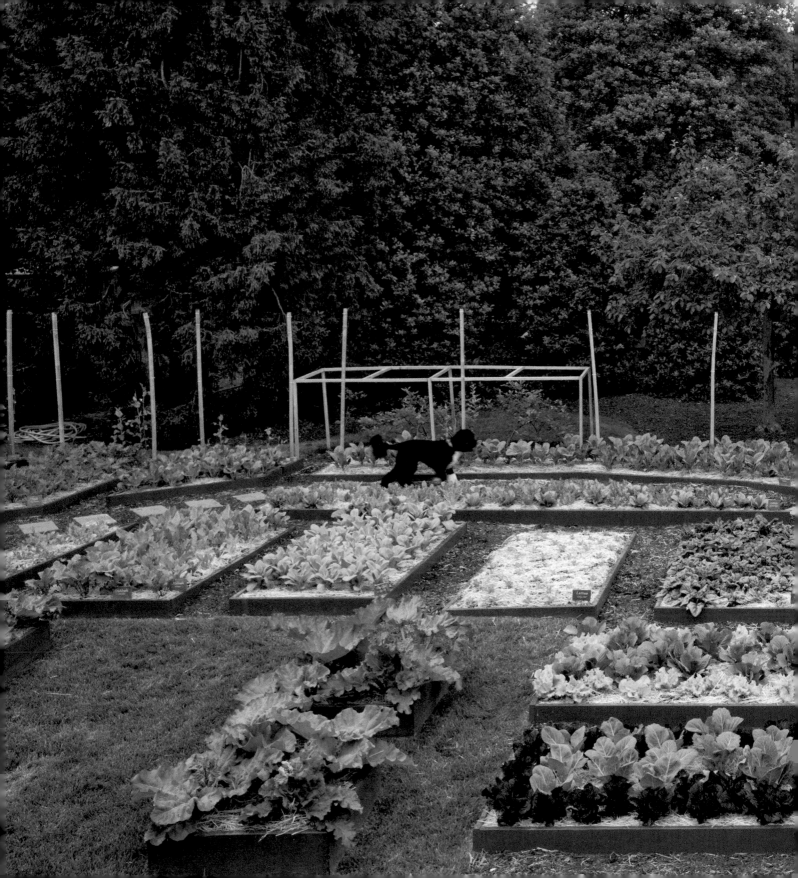

THE SPRING GARDEN 2011

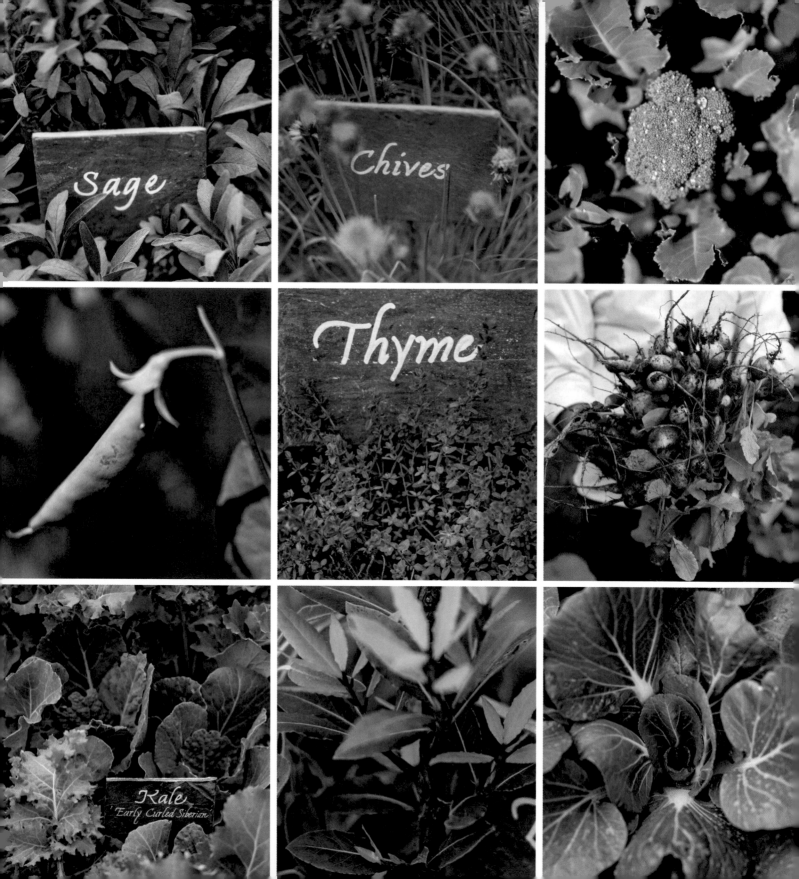

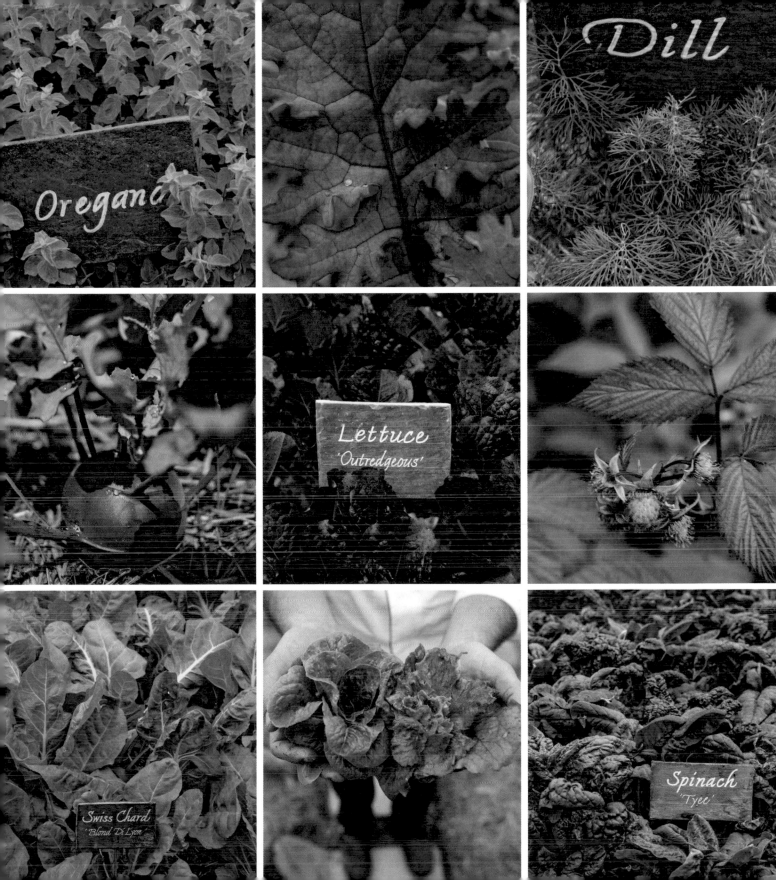

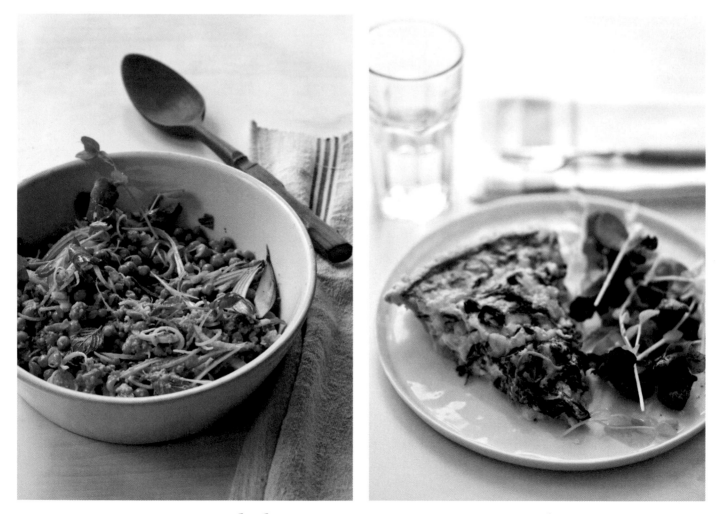

spring pea salad
page 221

spinach pie
page 222

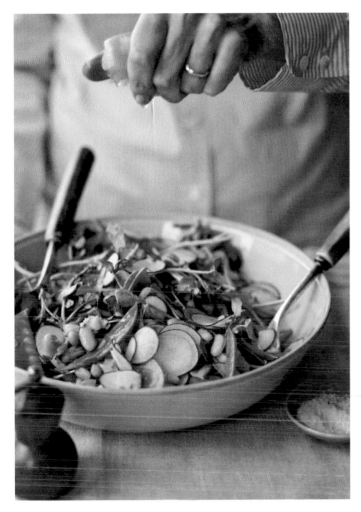

white bean salad
page 225

rhubarb strawberry
crumble pie
page 226

FINAL THOUGHTS ON SPRING

A garden in spring is not just the starting point for growing fresh, nutritious, delicious food. It can also be the beginning of new experiences and new lessons about where our food comes from and how it affects our health.

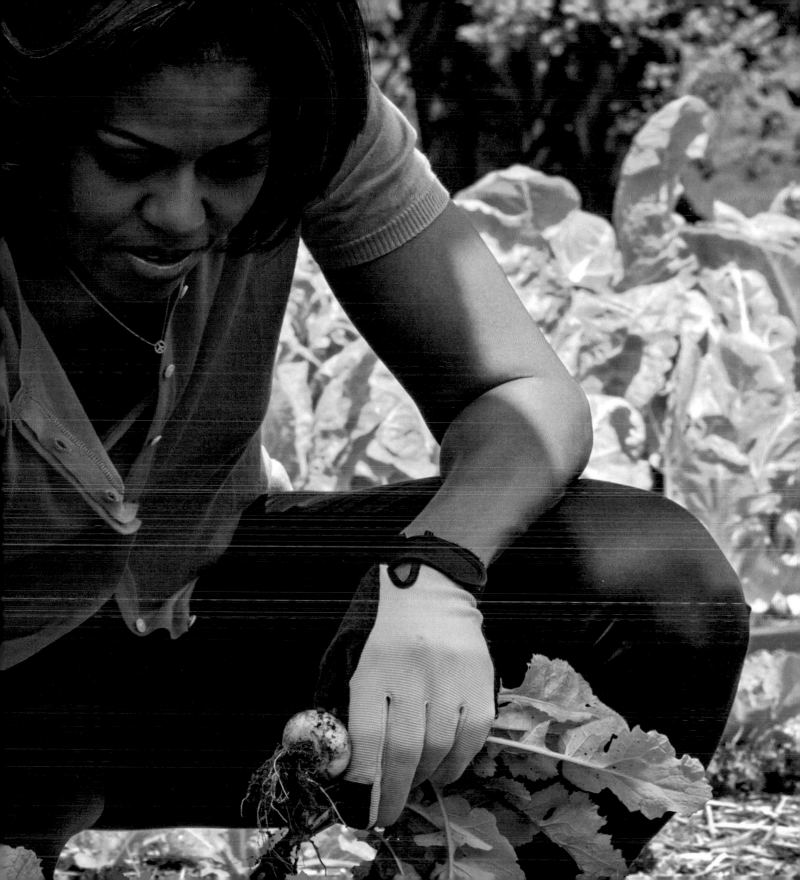

Summer

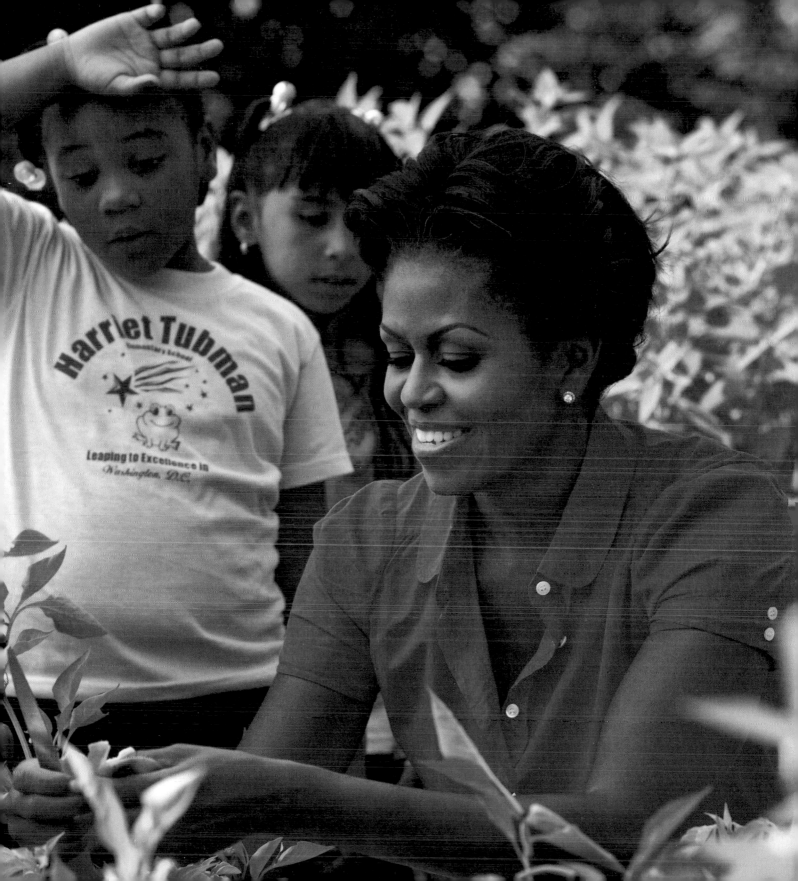

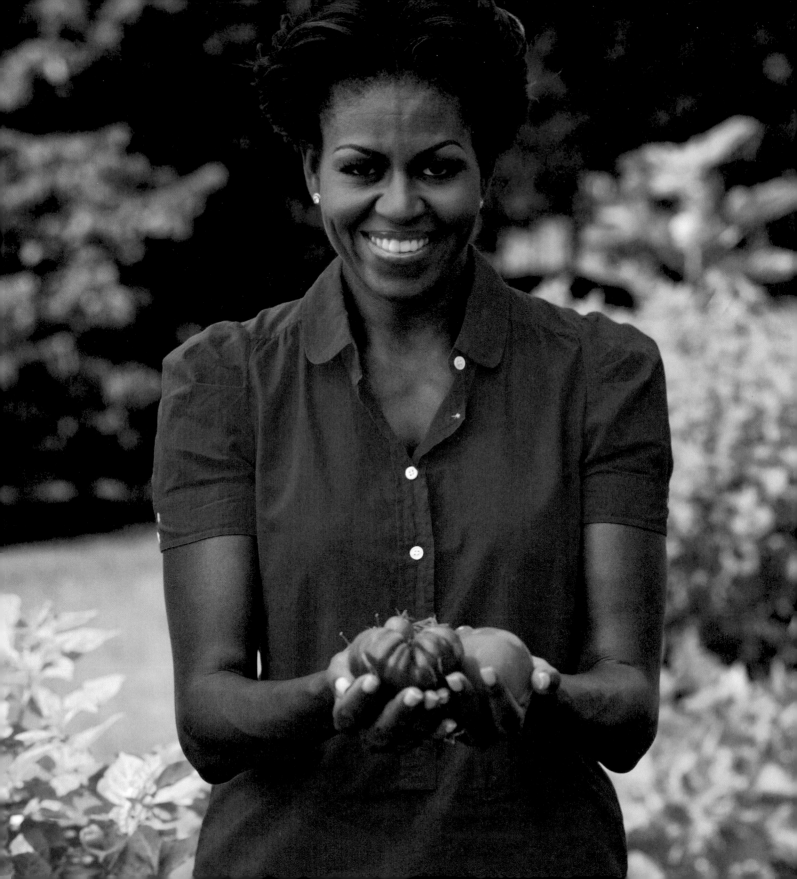

SUMMER: GROWING GARDENS AND STRONGER COMMUNITIES

In our garden, summer is a season of growth, with
tiny seedlings sprouting into lush plants and new
vegetables ripening every day. But gardens also grow so
much more. They bring people together—family, friends,
neighbors, even strangers united by their desire for a
successful harvest. And they give us a chance to work
with, and learn from, each other, reminding us of
all we have in common and helping us grow stronger,
more connected communities.

In the summer, Washington, D.C., is a tough town for a garden. The weather here can be brutal. In 2011 alone, we had a summer drought and a heat wave, with temperatures hovering around 100 degrees. Then we had an earthquake and, four days later, a hurricane, which was followed by a tropical rainstorm that caused serious flooding, including on the South Lawn of the White House.

By the end of the summer, our corn had been flattened, except for a few stalks that we coaxed back up, and our tomatoes were largely gone. But the Seminole squash plants had miraculously not just survived, they had taken over, growing not only in their own bed but into the surrounding beds as

THE LITTLE FIG TREE THAT COULD

Along with our Thomas Jefferson bed, we also planted a Thomas Jefferson fig tree. It was just one foot tall, and we planted it in the middle of the mint. By midsummer, it was growing rapidly, and the garden team was hoping that we would have figs by fall.

We checked on the tree regularly, and one Thursday afternoon Sam Kass went to see how it was doing. When he arrived at the garden, he discovered that the tree was gone. Not a trace of it was left. Sam had a moment of panic, and as he frantically looked around for some sign of where it had gotten to, he caught sight of our compost bin. On a whim, he raced over and opened it up, and there, lying on top of all the other compost, was the fig tree. A well-meaning volunteer must have thought it was a weed and pulled it, roots and all, from the bed.

Sam lifted it out of the bin and carefully replanted and watered it. But for the rest of the year, that fig tree was not happy. It lost its leaves early, as if it were holding a grudge. But it survived three massive winter snowstorms, and the next year it started to grow. Then, in the scorching heat of July 2011, the fig tree went crazy. In two months, it shot up until it was taller

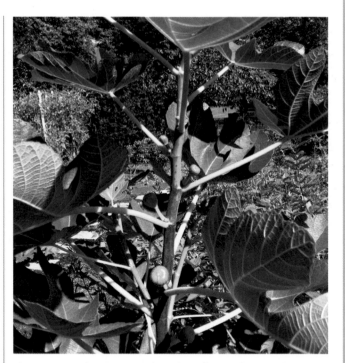

than me, and it sprouted its first figs. The weather kept the figs from fully ripening, but we loved seeing them thrive. And we're all keeping our fingers crossed for a bountiful fig harvest this year.

well. I don't know if it was the Three Sisters planting method or the miracle of Jefferson Keel's blessing at the planting, but those squash flourished despite their circumstances. Looking at them, you'd think every day had been sunny and 72 degrees.

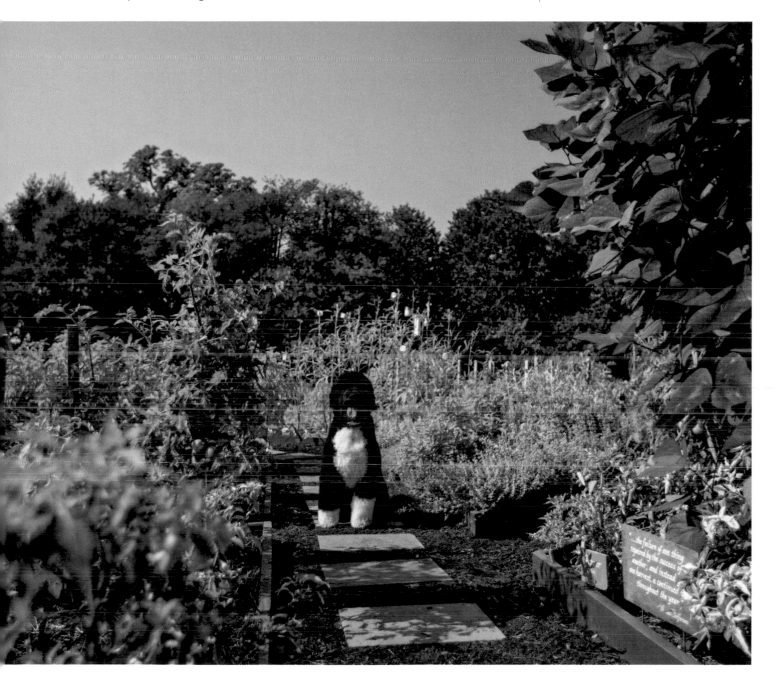

How Our Gardens Grow Stronger Communities

Kids often ask me, "Do you plant your garden by yourself?" and I say that I'm grateful that I don't have to, because our garden is so big that if I had to do it all by myself, it would never get done. Our garden, I tell them, is a community effort.

I am amazed and delighted at how many people think of this garden as *their* garden. The National Park Service gardeners take pride in the quality of the soil and the health of the plants. The chefs make lists of what they would like to grow and wander down with their bowls and baskets to harvest from the garden's beds. White House staffers volunteer their time many mornings before work. And then there are all the schoolchildren who have passed through, helping us plant and harvest the garden and enjoying what they've sown and picked. Without anyone expecting it, our garden has become a community garden, connecting people from all different backgrounds, ages, and walks of life. We all share in its care and in its success; and here in this garden, each of us, in

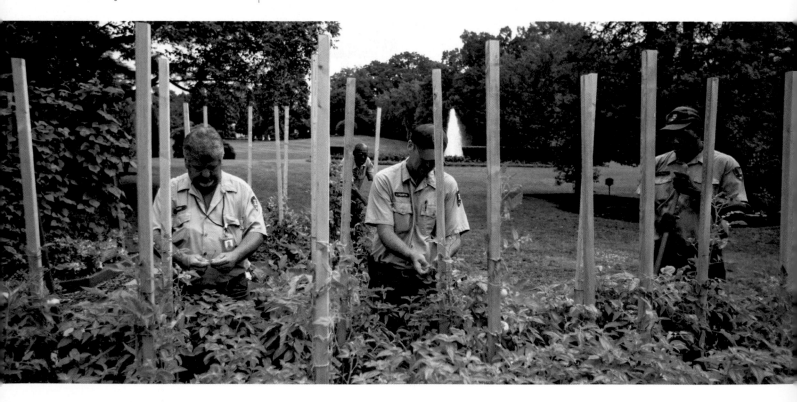

our own way, has been able to put down roots.

We're seeing this same phenomenon all across the country. People are working together to reclaim empty land and grow crops in their neighborhoods. Senior citizens are gardening with local youth in community gardens. Some gardeners grow produce for food banks, to ensure that everyone in their community has access to fresh, healthy food. Altogether there are about eighteen thousand community gardens in the United States and Canada. Here are some of their stories.

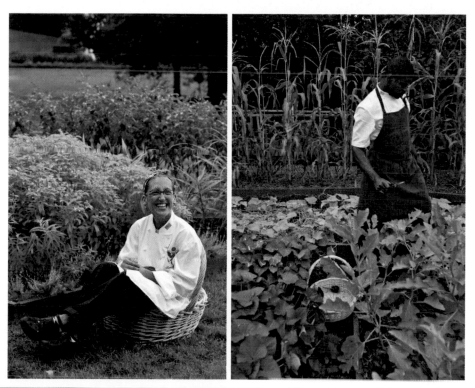

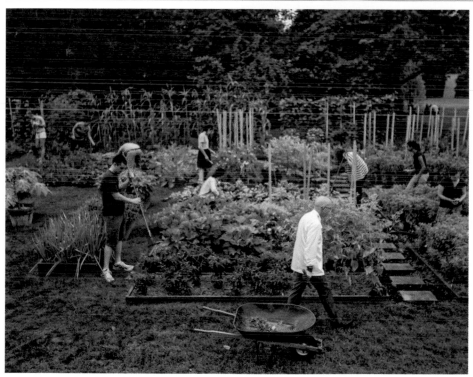

THE WHITE HOUSE TEAM
We had hoped that our garden would help build community among the many people who work in the White House. Volunteer mornings in the garden help do just that.

City Gardens, HOUSTON, TEXAS

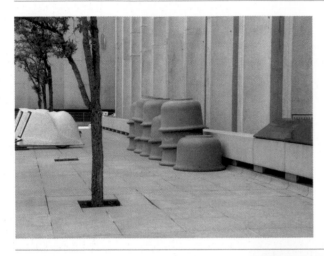

For years, the only thing outside the Bob Lanier Public Works Building in Houston, Texas, was concrete. That changed in June 2010, when landscape architect Keiji Asakura, Urban Harvest Director Mark Bowen, and Laura Spanjian, Houston's Director of Sustainability, joined together to establish a container garden in the heart of the city's downtown. Within three weeks, Houston's Parks Department had donated thirty-four planting containers; Keep Houston Beautiful had offered up soil and tools; and local nurseries had donated plants, such as okra, tomatoes, sweet potatoes, and squash, which thrive in the heavy summer heat.

When planting day arrived, about two hundred people, including Mayor Annise Parker, showed up to help dig in the dirt. Today, seventy-five people who work in the Bob Lanier building devote time to maintaining this garden. Tambri Elkins is one of those employees.

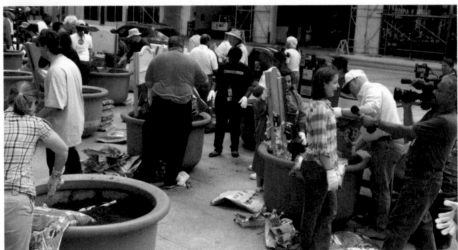

"By nature and by nurture I am a gardener. I didn't know about this project; I literally stumbled onto the containers and the soil and the plants as I was leaving the building for a lunch date. I looked around and canceled my lunch. It was so forward thinking for our city, and it fit my philosophy of 'If you are going to grow something, make sure your time is spent on plants that give you something back.' But this garden offered more. The ability to de-stress during the day, to unwind with the sun on my back and my hands in the earth, to smell wet soil, and to feel the texture of each plant on my fingertips was too tantalizing to

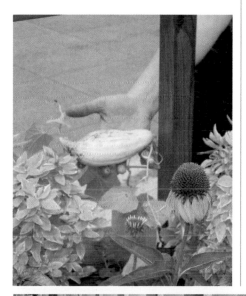

CITY GARDENS
A concrete landscape is transformed by simple containers growing bountiful plants, each cared for by volunteers from a single floor of an office building.

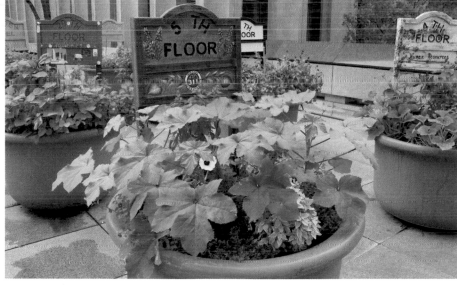

ignore. And I could be out there in the blazing Houston sun with like-minded individuals. How could I say no?

"The garden's organization also appealed to me. Each floor of the Lanier building had adopted a container; we picked a coordinator for the floor and found volunteers to plant and tend and water what was grown. We paired enthusiastic novice gardeners with more experienced ones, so there could be teaching and learning.

"I grew up in Southern California at a time when it was all strawberry fields, artichoke plants, avocado trees, Concord grapes, and citrus farming. Everyone had gardens and small orchards that were places to play, dream, and explore. At night, my family sat around the kitchen table looking at seed catalogs, heatedly discussing what to plant. As a child, gardens gave me shade, limbs to climb up to the sky, even green apples to entice a few horses that in my imagination carried me to far-away lands. The sap from fig trees, which works like itching powder, was payback to siblings. I remember picking small, red tomatoes, heated from the sun, and popping them in my mouth to quench my thirst. I remember sitting under the fruit trees staring at all the neat garden rows, watching for the first sign of life, dreading all the weeds that had to be pulled, and waiting for the exact day when a fruit or vegetable was at its peak for picking. All these memories come back to me in our small, urban container garden.

"Our city garden is a lesson that anyone can grow food with a minimal amount of space, time, money, and energy. In these containers, we produce not only sustenance but also pride and confidence. The gardeners meet people who work in the same building, who we may have passed for years in hallways, but we never knew their names. And whenever I'm in the garden, someone always walks by and asks, 'What are you growing?'"

—TAMBRI ELKINS

"To me, gardens are small reminders of all the wonders of the universe."
—TAMBRI ELKINS,
Senior Human Resources Specialist, City of Houston, and Veteran Gardener

The Readington Community Garden,

READINGTON TOWNSHIP, NEW JERSEY

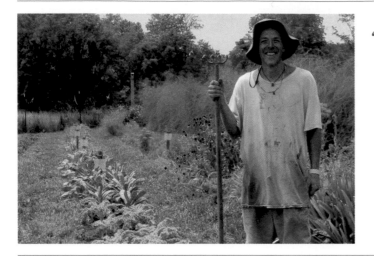

"People are constantly bringing their kids to help. I like seeing moms and dads walk down the rows with their children. It's a teaching sort of thing as well as a food garden."

—DAN ALLEN,
Garden Cofounder

"I grew up on a farm, but I was never into gardening. Then, in my twenties, I was working at a soul-crushing corporate job and I started planting stuff as an escape. I discovered that I enjoyed it, and it led me to regrow my own life. I started taking ecology classes and quit my job. I worked on organic farms; then I started teaching high school chemistry and doing some farming on the side.

"Where we live is the edge of suburban sprawl in New Jersey. My mom, Julia, had been the town mayor for years and she has worked hard to help protect farmland around here. But in our town, most people have lawns and not much time to put in a garden patch. I have a plot in my own yard, and I had worked on my parents' garden, often selling what we grew at a stand at the end of the driveway. But I got it into my head that we would really benefit from a community garden.

"My friend Chip Shepherd, a great middle school science teacher, wanted to help. We chose a site that was a third of an acre. We put an ad in the township newsletter and the local paper wrote a front-page story on us. Fifty people came to our first meeting. Now we don't advertise at all; it's just word of mouth. We have everyone from people in their seventies to toddlers who come to work on the garden. Some people have been growing things for years; some have never set a plant in the ground. We had one woman who started putting in all our strawberry plants upside down. We learned pretty quickly to pair the novices with people who have more of a clue about what to do

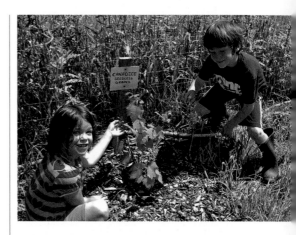

in a garden. And it's all worked out.

"We meet up every Saturday morning. It's amazing how much twenty to fifty relatively unskilled people can do to clean up a garden. It's completely weeded and whipped into shape in about two hours. We started our garden with basically no rules. You can come during the week or on the weekends; there are no assigned

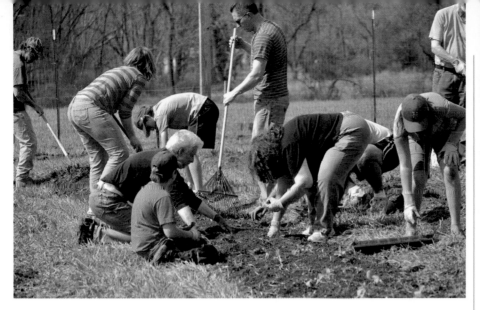

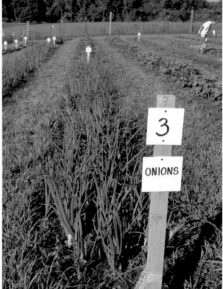

work hours; and there's no lock on our fence. About a third of the people come every week, another third come every couple of weeks, and a third of the people are new or hardly ever come. We don't have any annual fee either. Many families contribute $20 a year toward expenses, but not all.

"Throughout the season, we divide up our harvest completely on the honor system. When the vegetables are harvested, we call out on Saturday mornings what is ready for harvest, from kale to collards to strawberries or eggplant. People know how much they have contributed to the garden and take from what's ready accordingly. And each year, we learn something about planting. In 2010, our tomatoes kept running out, so the next year, we planted twice as many of them. We've also planted more than twenty fruit and nut seedlings to start an orchard.

"There's nothing like being outside on a hot and humid July morning in New Jersey to make you aware of a whole other world. And in our garden we are trying to conserve our connections to each other—the bonds of our community—by working and talking together in a shared meaningful endeavor.

"In all of this, I'd like to think that we are succeeding. We're growing good vegetables and a good community at the same time."

—Dan Allen

"There is nothing like the taste of food fresh from the ground. If you harvest a potato and cook it the same day, it always tastes sweeter."

—Chip Shepherd,
Garden Cofounder

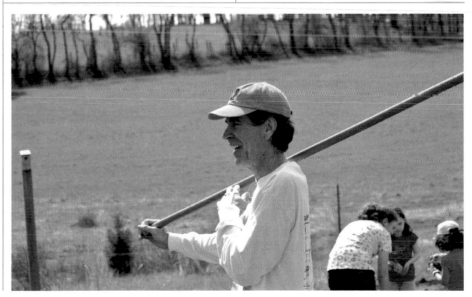

P-Patch, SEATTLE, WASHINGTON

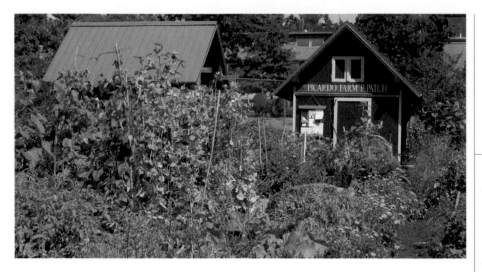

In 1973, the city of Seattle, Washington, launched its first community garden at a farm owned by the Picardo family (the P in "P-Patch"). The plot had no water lines; gardeners actually had to fill up milk jugs and other containers to carry water to their patches. P-Patch nearly failed in the early 1980s when Seattle experienced a serious economic downturn. But the gardeners persevered, winning national awards, and P-Patch became the largest municipal community gardening program in the country.

Today, there are seventy-six P-Patch gardens spread across Seattle, on twenty-three acres, with forty-seven hundred gardeners. Some gardeners live below the poverty line, and some have visited a food bank in the last year. Almost a third of the gardeners get a majority of their produce from their garden plots in the spring and summer months, and about a quarter do so in the winter. About a third of the gardeners also donate some of their harvest to food banks and feeding centers: 20,889 pounds of fresh produce were given away in 2010.

Michael and Rebecca McGoodwin have been growing produce in their P-Patch plot since 2003.

"Rebecca comes from a long line of farmers and gardeners, while I had spent years trying to avoid getting my hands dirty in the garden. But since we started, I've been coming up to full steam. Most people would probably want a garden on their own property, but P-Patch gardening offers a special atmosphere and advantages not found on private land. Beyond being able to share communal resources such as tools and compost, we get to know our fellow gardeners and can chat over the crop rows with casual passersby. We also have many chances to get together down at the 'Patch' with fellow gardeners for informal potluck suppers where we exchange notes on what plants are working well.

"There are frustrations, however. We lost potatoes and beets in 2008 to an invasion of rats (neighboring gardeners lost sugar snap peas), and in 2006, in part because there are no fences, eight prized winter squashes that we had babied all through the hot summer were stolen. But we have persevered.

"While store-bought vegetables are getting more and more expensive, the primary benefit of raising your own vegetables is the deep satisfaction that comes from returning to the basics of tilling the soil, raising the crops, and thereby addressing our most primitive needs for sustenance. Getting to the P-Patch can also present a welcome respite from the urban rat race and seem like a little trip to the country."

—MICHAEL MCGOODWIN

Rainbow Beach Park, CHICAGO, ILLINOIS

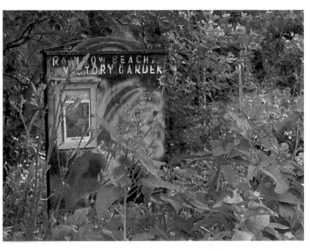

"Before or after gardening, I love wandering around other gardeners' plots and admiring their beautiful flowers. Every color you can imagine is represented somewhere in the garden."
—DREA EISENBERG
Recent Rainbow Beach Gardener

Rainbow Beach Park was named for the U.S. Army's Forty-second Rainbow Division, formed during World War I by soldiers who were hastily called up from twenty-six states and the District of Columbia. Douglas MacArthur, then a colonel, coined its name: He described the unit as stretching like a rainbow, covering the country from one end of the sky to the other. During World War II, Chicagoans covered much of this parkland with a victory garden, and the Rainbow Beach Victory Garden remains in that location to this day.

It is the oldest community garden in the city, with seventy years of mulch having been laid down on its beds. The garden holds more than forty large individual plots, most bordered by bright flowers. There are vegetables and even fruit trees growing in between grass walkways. Each plot stays with its gardener until he or she retires or moves on, and many have been cultivated by the same gardener for decades. A recent Rainbow Beach gardener, Drea Eisenberg, explains, "It is so special tilling the same soil that someone tilled sixty or seventy years ago."

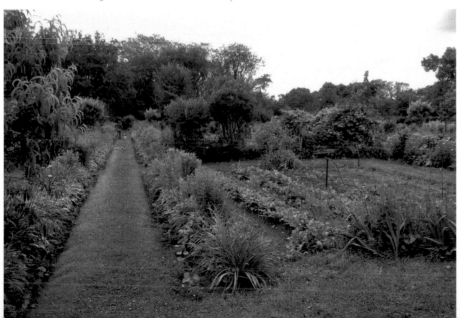

NURTURING THE PAST
About forty gardeners have plots in Rainbow Beach Park. It blooms with summer vegetables, flowers, and native prairie plants.

Gardens of Service, WINSTON-SALEM, NORTH CAROLINA

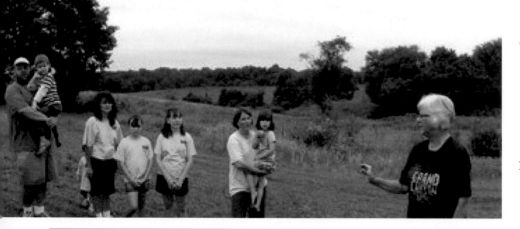

> *"The mission and message of this garden is what we grow, we give back."*
>
> —ELLEN KIRBY,
> Betty and Jim Holmes Food Bank Garden

The only known, well-documented colonial community garden in America was the "Garden at Bethabara," planted in 1753 in Winston-Salem, North Carolina, by Protestant Moravian immigrants. Today the city of Winston-Salem is blooming with community gardens of all shapes and sizes—and many of these are gardens of service—gardens cultivated to help those in need. Volunteers are starting community gardens for recovering addicts, physically and emotionally challenged children, and residents who live in Habitat for Humanity houses.

A garden of service was also started at Kimberley Park Elementary School in 2010. Here six fourth-grade girls and their mothers began working in two small plots to grow tomatoes, squash, cucumbers, peppers, beans, and okra. During those hours of planting, weeding, and watering, they talked, listened, and laughed, sharing stories and advice and reminding us that gardens don't just connect us to our land and our food, but to each other.

The Betty and Jim Holmes Food Bank Garden is another good example of a community garden devoted to serving others. At three acres, this garden is one of the largest gardens in the city, sitting just three miles from the city's downtown. The garden has been in operation for fifteen years, and every vegetable, melon, and herb that is harvested from its soil is donated to the Second Harvest Food Bank.

Today, one of the lead gardeners is Ellen Kirby, a Winston-Salem native who returned home after living in New York City for forty years.

"I first got interested in gardening because I got tired of traveling and staying in hotels for my job. I saw the inside of airports and planes and I wanted to be outside. My church

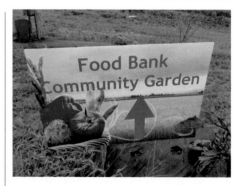

in Brooklyn, New York, had a garden, and the people who had been taking care of it were moving, so I volunteered. I discovered that I loved plants. Some mornings, I'd head over to the garden at 5 a.m. so that I could get my 'gardening fix' for the week before I boarded a plane.

"Eventually, after turning the churchyard garden into a community garden, I realized that this was what I should be doing full-time. I got a job at the Brooklyn Botanic Garden

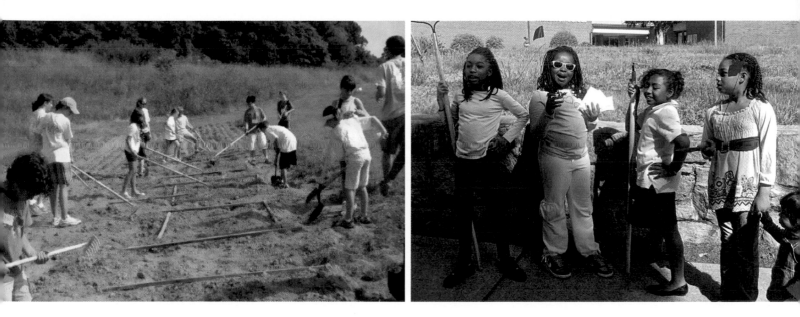

GROWING FOR OTHERS
Volunteers at the Betty and Jim Holmes Food Bank Garden prepare the soil (above). *Kimberley Park School gardeners are all smiles* (above, right).

and worked to start GreenBridge, the botanic garden's community environmental horticulture program, and from there I also became a president of the American Community Gardening Association. I came home to Winston-Salem to 'retire' and ended up right back in the garden.

"I love the mission and the message of this garden. What we grow, we give back. All our produce is given to Second Harvest, the regional food bank, which serves eighteen North Carolina counties. Each garden harvest is transported right away to participating local grocery stores, where it is kept in their refrigerated sections until it is picked up by Second Harvest's refrigerated trucks. Very fragile items, like lettuce, are delivered directly to local soup kitchens. It's a big community working together—gardeners, merchants, truck drivers, everyone with one goal: to get the freshest food to the people who need it the most.

"Our garden succeeds because of the dedication of our volunteers. Good people make a great garden, and we are cultivating people as much as plants. There are twenty to thirty core people, primarily from Centenary United Methodist Church, our local sponsor, who come every one or two weeks. Beyond that, it has become a spot for local volunteer groups to donate their time and muscle. On a given morning, members of a synagogue might arrive with fifty volunteers. Nearby Wake Forest University brought fifty entering business school students to work in the garden one fall and returned with twenty in the spring. On a cold January day, the Winston-Salem State University's women's softball team cleared the fields to prepare for spring planting. Churches, garden clubs, and schoolteachers and their students also come to help. The result is that we harvest anywhere from five thousand to nine thousand pounds of food a year. This garden is the only source of regular, fresh produce for many people in our region, and we get joy from being able to share with them our harvest of fresh, local food."

—ELLEN KIRBY

New Roots Community Farm, SAN DIEGO, CALIFORNIA

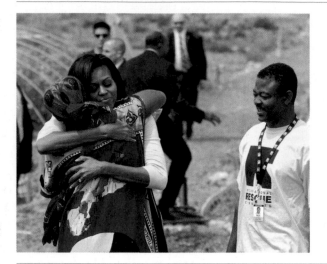

"I get food from the garden, and it connects me with my family because I grew up on a small farm in Zimbabwe."

—TSITSI MUTSETA,
New Roots Gardener

In San Diego, I visited a new generation of community gardeners at the New Roots Community Farm, where the gardeners are immigrants from around the world. Although they hailed from different countries, they all recognized that many recent immigrants like themselves were struggling to get by on tight budgets and were skipping fresh fruits and vegetables and settling for fast food instead. As a result, many of them were suffering from high cholesterol and high blood pressure.

Together, they resolved to do something about this, and they decided to start by growing their own garden. After two years of fundraising and organizing, gardeners from countries across the globe, including Uganda, Kenya, Vietnam, Mexico, and Guatemala, broke ground together.

At first, they weren't sure how people from so many different countries would get along—especially since the garden had only two hoses to share and the farmers often didn't speak the same language. But their enthusiasm and determination drew them together. And day by day, little by little, neighbors started sharing their vegetables. They started exchanging recipes. And they started recognizing the hopes and dreams they held in common: to make a home for themselves here in America, to keep their families healthy, and to give their kids a better life.

During the height of growing season, these farmers harvest about a thousand pounds of produce a week. These crops provide both fresh food for their families and a chance to make an income—the produce is sold at a local farmers' market and to several local restaurants. The New Roots Community Farm has also given these gardeners something more: a sense of community and a chance to regrow their lives.

Embracing Khadija Musame, a refugee from Somalia. Bilal Muya looks on (above). Speaking with Tsitsi Mutseta, originally from Zimbabwe (opposite).

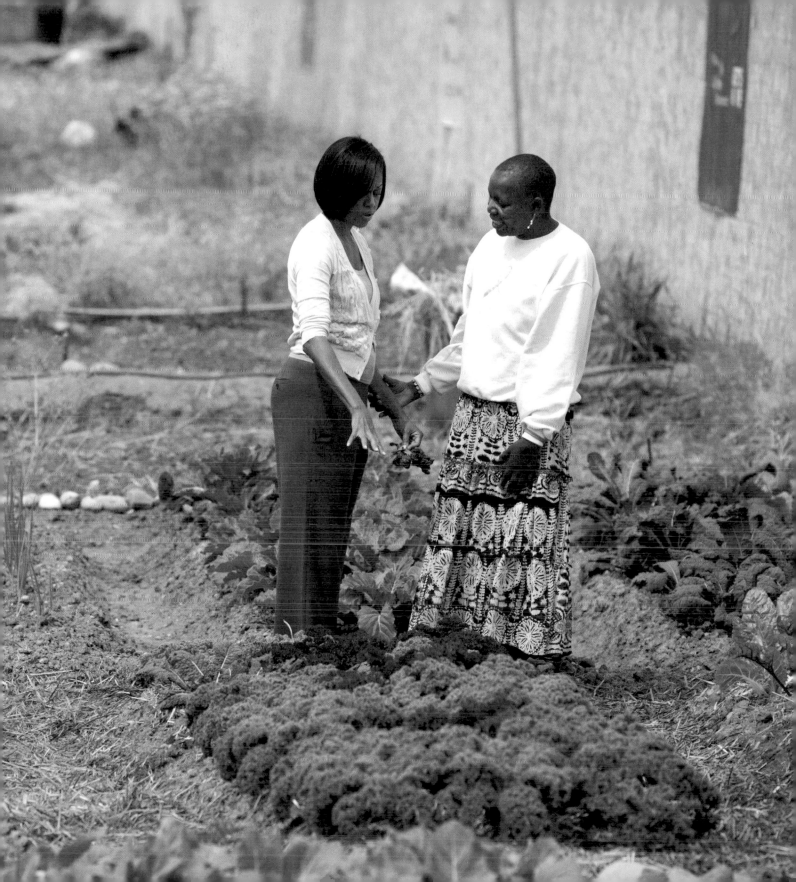

Growing a Community Garden

If you would like to be part of a community garden, you can start by going to the American Community Garden Association's website, www.community garden.org, where you can type in your zip code and find listings, descriptions, and contact information for community gardens nearby. If there aren't any gardens in your area, the association also provides a detailed guide on how to start your own, covering everything from leases to site selection to insurance.

"Every person should live within a certain distance of the opportunity to grow something," says Ben Helphand, director of NeighborSpace, which helps locate and preserve community garden land in Chicago. Helphand and other experienced gardeners offer the following suggestions for budding community gardeners:

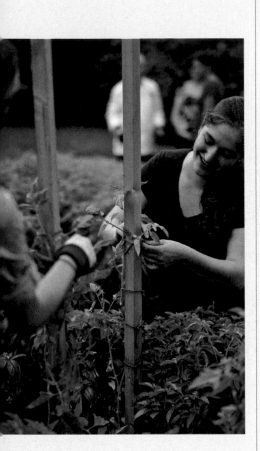

It all starts with the land. It's important to select a site that is protected, whether by a city or county agency, a social service institution, or a private owner. Many communities have local land trusts that help secure gardening sites not just for a few years but for decades.

The community comes first. Everyone involved needs to have a clear idea of what the garden is for. Will each gardener grow his or her own produce on individual plots, or will everyone pool their resources to create a common garden? Should there be only vegetables, or should there be flowers too? Who will be in charge of assigning the plots? Some gardeners prefer to have basic rules or even written bylaws and garden officers who oversee the garden.

Ask for help. Whenever people are asked why they don't volunteer, the number one reason is that no one has asked them to help. Many community gardeners find that social media, such as Facebook, is a great way to draw volunteers, and weekly or monthly e-mails keep everyone connected. Telephone calls or posting information and sign-up sheets on garden bulletin boards work well too. Gardeners looking to troubleshoot a problem in their garden can find help on community garden forums, like the one maintained by the American Community Gardening Association or the local department of agriculture's extension service. And affiliating your garden with a church, school, or senior center is also a good way to link your garden to an existing community.

Start out with a manageable plan. Many community gardens fail because they overreach and neglect the basics: Start small, have access to water and compost, and build good soil. (See page 58 for additional tips on starting a garden.)

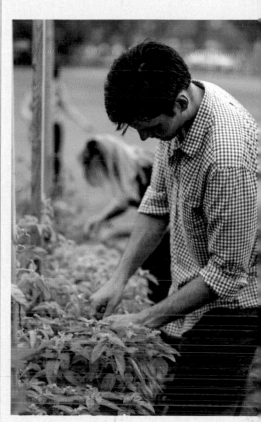

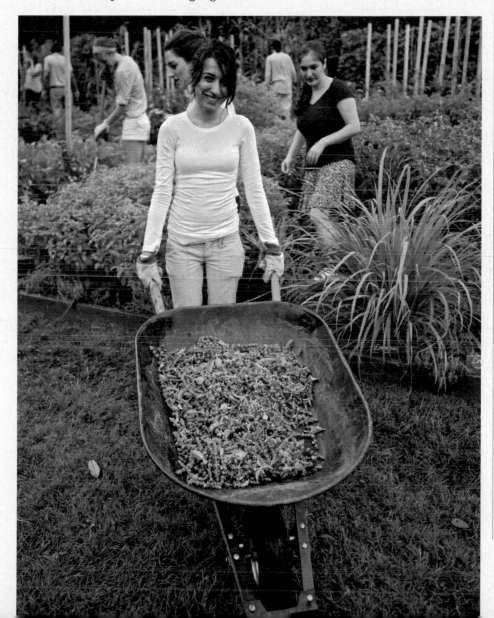

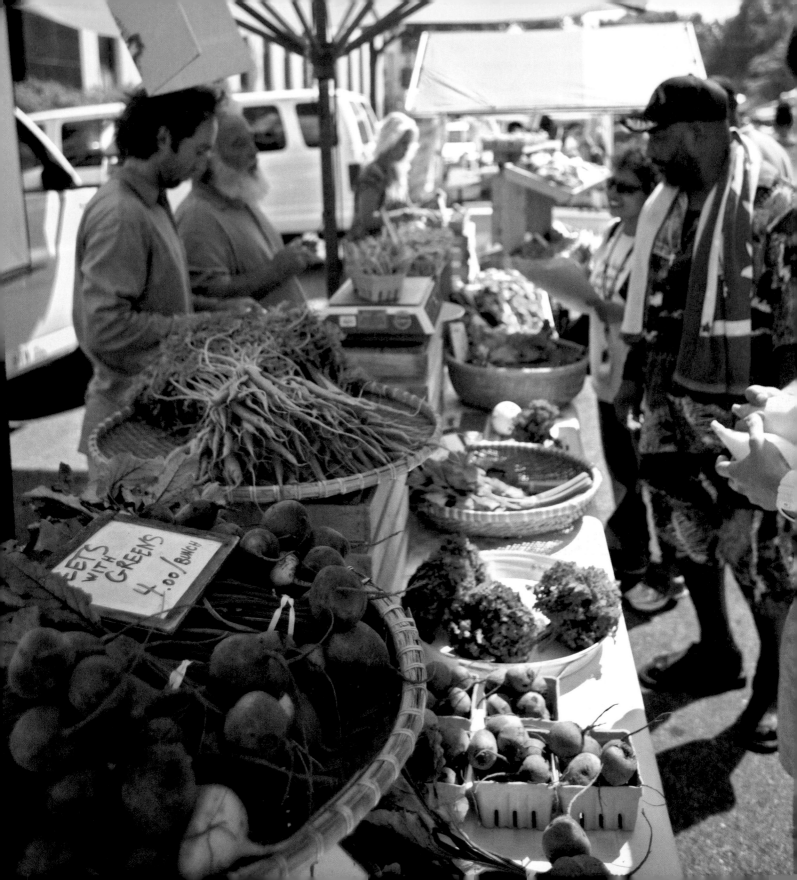

Farmers' Markets: Another Kind of Garden Community

Even if you don't have a garden, you can still be part of a garden community and share in what is garden grown by buying your produce from farmers' markets, places where local growers sell their products. There are more than seven thousand farmers' markets nationwide, and many of them offer prices that are competitive with those of supermarkets; many also accept food stamps.

Farmers' markets offer us a chance to know some of the people who grow our food and to taste a fresh-picked harvest—no shovel, hoe, or gardening gloves required. Farmers' markets can also be a great way to bring nutritious food to underserved communities. And these markets often become tight-knit communities of their own as growers and customers come together week after week, buying and selling fresh food and sharing recipes and casual conversation.

One of the first farmers' markets in Washington, D.C., was started by Thomas Jefferson, who would ask his maître d' to go out to the market and buy fresh produce for his guests. When I arrived in the White House, I decided that I wanted to bring a farmers' market to the neighborhood. Back home in Chicago, farmers' markets had been a great way for my family to find fresh produce and learn about healthy eating, and I wanted others to have that experience as well.

But while it had taken us only a couple of months to build a garden, it took much longer to bring in a market. We couldn't do it at the White House itself. As my husband joked with a group of reporters, "We're trying to figure out, can we get a little farmers' market outside the White House? I'm not going to have all of you just tromping around inside, but right outside the White House—that is a win-win situation."

People were excited about the idea, but the Washington, D.C., of 2009 was very different from the Washington, D.C., of 1801.

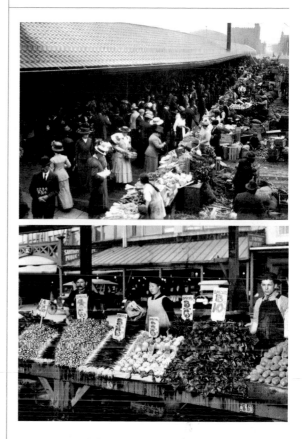

PIKE PLACE MARKET,
SEATTLE, WASHINGTON

Back in the early 1900s the city of Seattle sponsored a farmers' market as an experiment to help reduce the high cost of local produce. Via market stalls, farmers could sell directly to shoppers. The central rule for the market required that only food and food products "raised, produced, or manufactured" by the vendor could be sold. Pike Place has become a permanent fixture in Seattle.

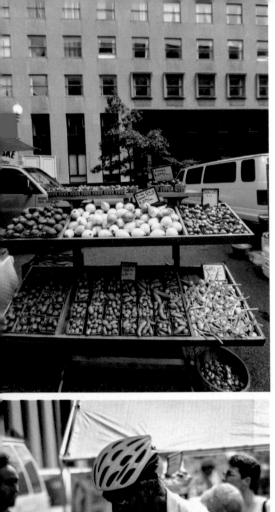

It took a lot of searching and many conversations with our local government, but eventually, we found a spot: Vermont Avenue, on a relatively quiet block right off Lafayette Park. On September 17, 2009, the Vermont Avenue Farmer's Market officially opened for business. At the grand opening, I had the chance to do some shopping and meet a few of the customers, some of whom work in nearby office buildings. The market is a place where they can slip out on a lunch break or stop and pick up something for dinner before they begin their commute home.

I try to get out of the bubble of the White House as often as possible. But it's not always easy, or even possible, for me to do my own food shopping, so it was fun for me to browse the rows of fresh fruits and vegetables. It was hard to pick among them—everything looked so enticing—but I finally settled on kale, cherry tomatoes, hot peppers, fingerling potatoes, and cheese, and we had a delicious vegetable ragout for dinner.

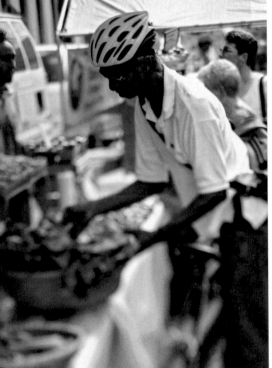

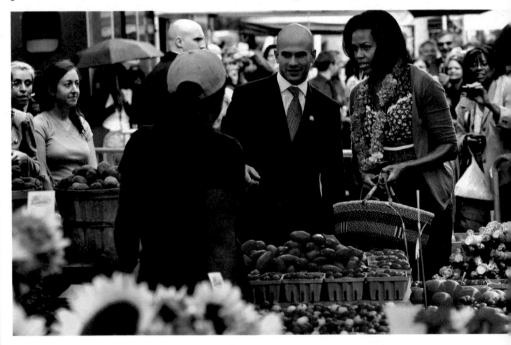

VERMONT AVENUE MARKET
Thomas Jefferson encouraged the growth of a farmers' market and sent his maître d' to shop there. In 2009, a new market opened near the White House.

SHOPPING FOR TOMATOES
Sam Kass and I shop at the market, which attracts mainly family farmers from the surrounding states and gives people who live and work downtown a chance to taste food straight from the fields or a local kitchen.

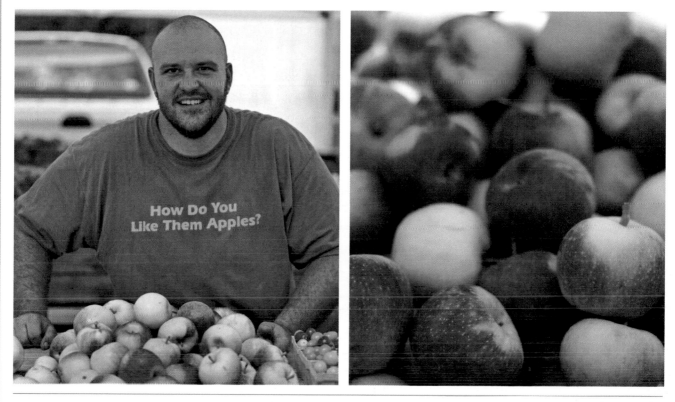

"My family has farmed the same land in West Virginia for five generations. My ancestors were the first people to grow fruit trees in Hampshire County before the Revolutionary War, and my great-grandfather picked our current spot because of its rocky soil, which adds a rich flavor to whatever fruits we grow. My grandfather still likes to pick our peaches.

"I always knew I'd come back to be a farmer, even when I did two combat tours with the Marines in Iraq. In between the sandstorms and patrols, I'd tell my buddies, many of whom were city boys, stories of life on the farm—the funny ones but also the hardships. It's not easy to have a few months of crop a year and make a decent profit. My U.S. Marine Corps buddies came up with the idea of selling what my family grows at farmers' markets. We had always just sold at our local fruit stand. I had never thought of farmers' markets and hadn't even been to one, but now I love it, even if I have to get up as early as 1:30 a.m. to make the drive into the city to be ready for some market openings. My buddies also told me to 'capture the taste in a jar.' So when I got home, we started making and selling preserved products, called Bigg Riggs.

"Along with our fruit trees, I've added a four-acre vegetable garden and a specially designed covered electric cart that I can use for picking, so I'm not constantly bending and squatting in the hot sun. It's hard work, but I wouldn't work at anything else. I feel like I can taste the history of my family and the land in every apple, peach, plum, pear, and cherry that we grow."
—CALVIN RIGGLEMAN

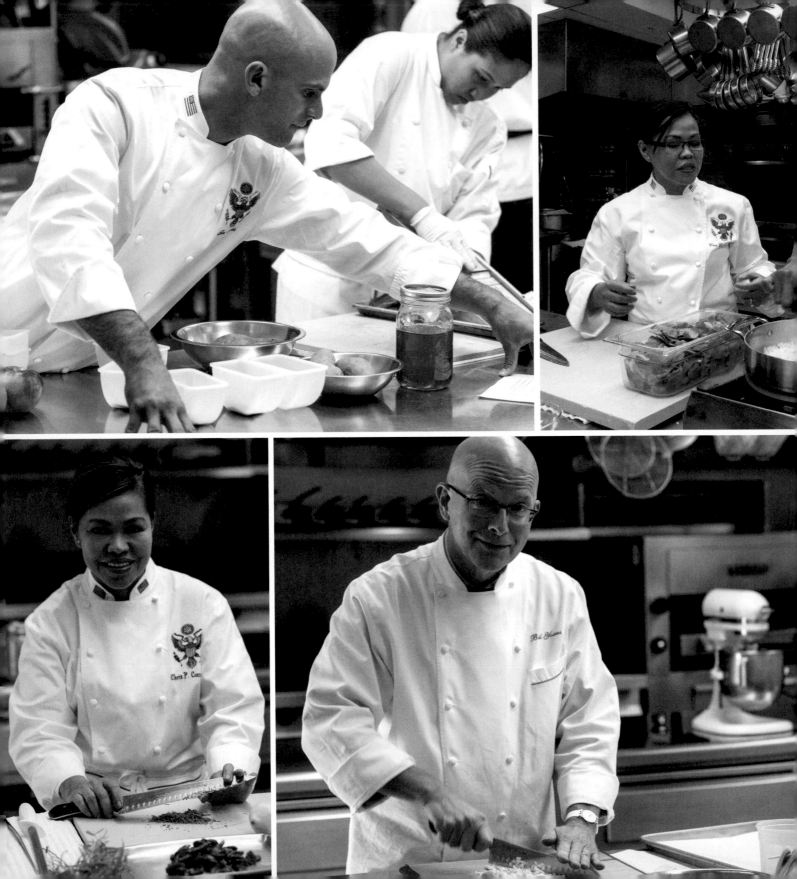

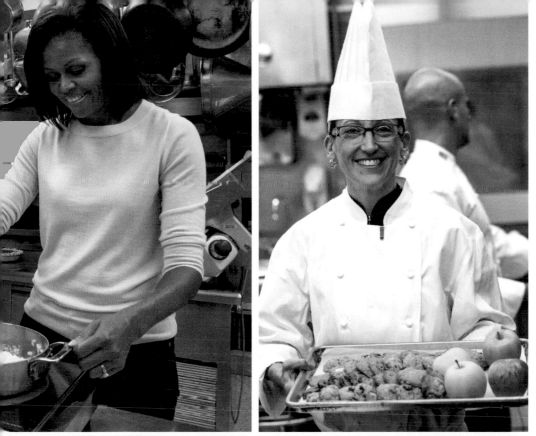

COMMUNITY IN THE KITCHEN

"We rely on a team effort to create our dishes; sometimes there are ten of us just in the pastry kitchen. And everyone has something to contribute." —Bill Yosses

"We learn from each other. We have so many chefs from different parts of the world, it's like musicians: Each plays a piece of classical music a little differently, and those differences help all of us. I've found that the best recipes are almost never secrets but are the ones that are shared among many chefs." —Cris Comerford

"The creative process is always enhanced by having a diverse set of minds and a diverse body of knowledge. It's been amazing to work with such incredible professionals who are cooking on such a big stage." —Sam Kass

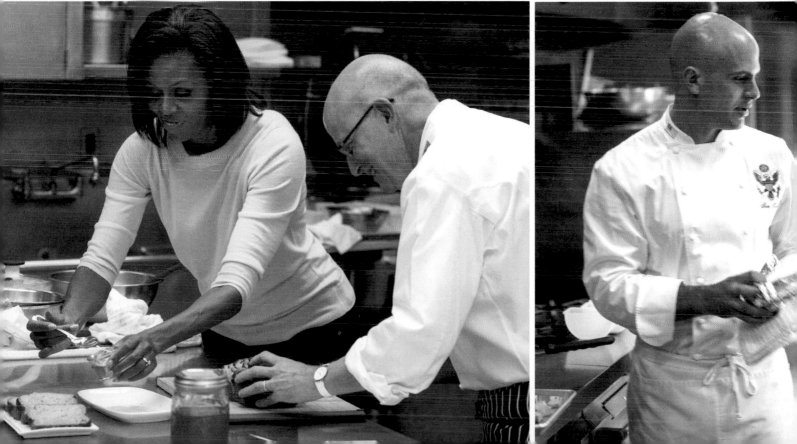

FINDING COMMUNITY IN THE KITCHEN GARDEN
Executive Pastry Chef Bill Yosses

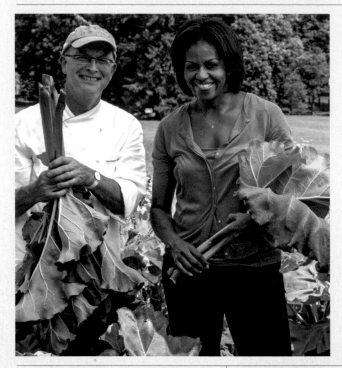

From the start, Mrs. Obama and everyone in the White House who was involved in the garden wanted to share it. We didn't want it to be our place; we wanted it to be everyone's place. After that first planting, I started leading a lot of the tours, taking kids around the drive past the upper South Lawn, and first to the beehive to talk about pollination. A few kids are scared of the bees, but most are fascinated, and few have ever seen a live hive before.

I also show them the herbs, and let them taste little bits, like the licorice flavor of anise hyssop or a bit of lemon verbena or cilantro.

A GATHERING PLACE

"The Kitchen Garden is about more than what grows here, although I am delighted whenever we have the chance to cook with our freshly harvested rhubarb stalks, as you can see above. The garden is also about learning and people and sharing. It is a welcoming place."
—Chef Bill

MANY HANDS

"Every Tuesday at 8:15 a.m., volunteers from across the White House come to help in the garden. It doesn't matter if you haven't gardened before—everyone is welcome, and anyone can learn."
—Chef Bill

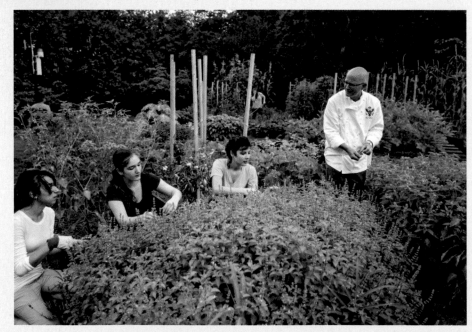

I like the fact that our garden is a hands-on, learning garden. Kids can sniff, they can taste, and they can break off a piece of herb and literally hold part of the garden in their hands. We stop by the Thomas Jefferson bed and talk about the importance of agriculture in American history, how growing food and eating well has been a tradition since our beginnings as a nation. We talk about growing a garden, about planting seasonally, about caring for the soil. For the little kids, the best part is the compost, where they can dig for worms with their hands. They love the idea that a lot of soil is worm poop.

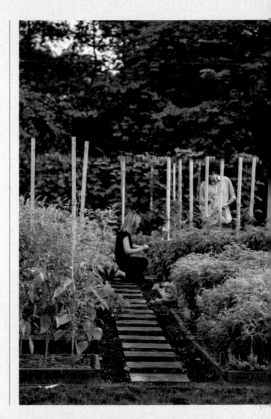

But we soon realized that kids weren't the only ones who wanted to see the garden. People who worked for the President in the White House and in its surrounding buildings were also eager for a relationship with the garden. They wanted to get their hands in it, literally. I sent out my first e-mail blast looking for volunteers in 2009. I was hoping to get twenty people who might be interested in weeding and doing some garden work early on a Tuesday morning. I got hundreds of replies. Some of the people had worked in community gardens before joining the White House as staff members. We have people who have studied environmental policy, agriculture, and food policy, and they come in gardening clothes, ready to work. We start just after the first planting in March and go into November. And every week, in rain or heat or cold, the roster is full.

The demand is so great that we usually have a new group of volunteers each week just so that we can make sure to include everyone who wants to help. Jim Adams and I give them a brief tutorial on how the garden is built and on weeding and watering, but everyone is a quick learner. You don't have to show them something twice.

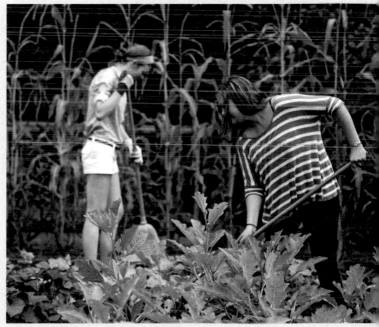

In the spring of 2010, I attended a big event on healthy eating, and I saw a woman in a military officer's uniform. She looked very familiar to me, and as we started speaking, I realized that she had been one of my garden volunteers. I hadn't known she was a military officer; she had simply shown up in work clothes like everyone else. I never cease to be amazed by the wonders, big and small, of this one garden.

THE 2011
Summer Garden
PLAN

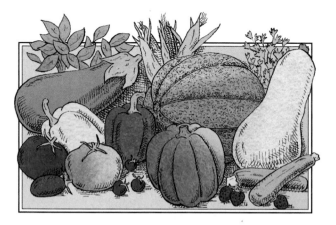

"Without anyone expecting it, our garden has become a community garden, connecting people from all different backgrounds, ages, and walks of life."

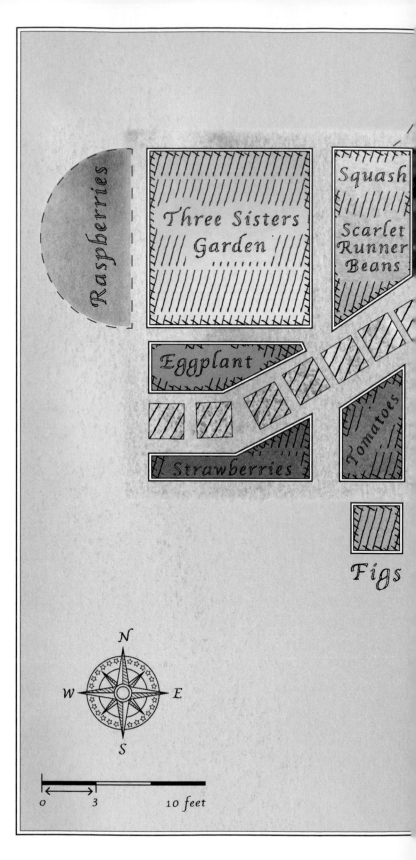

Raspberries

Three Sisters Garden

Squash

Scarlet Runner Beans

Eggplant

Strawberries

Tomatoes

Figs

N
W   E
S

0   3   10 feet

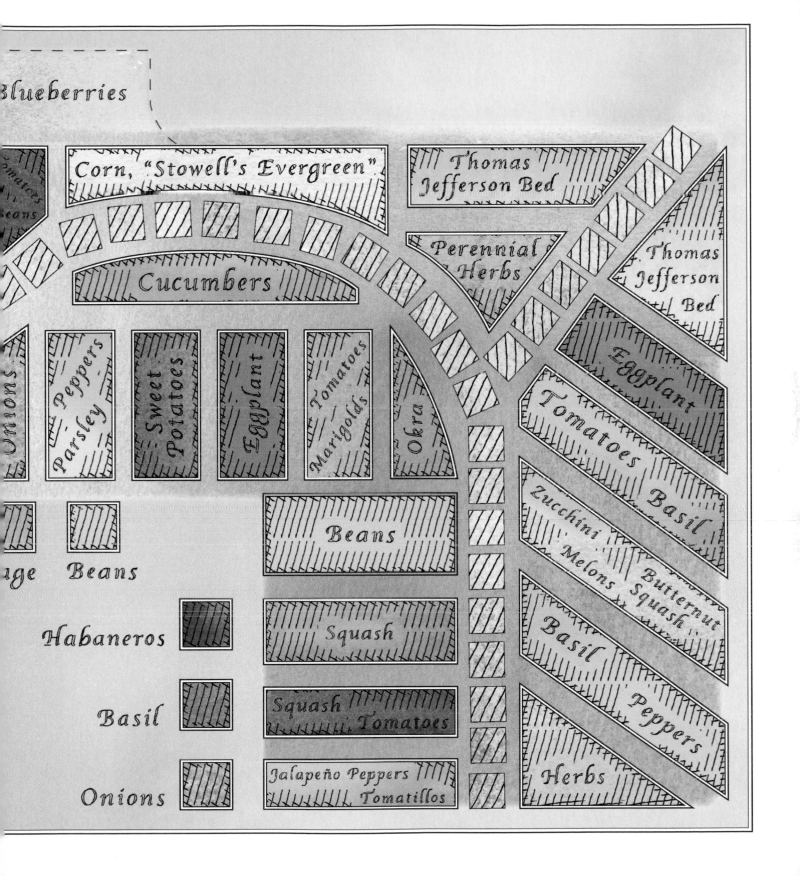

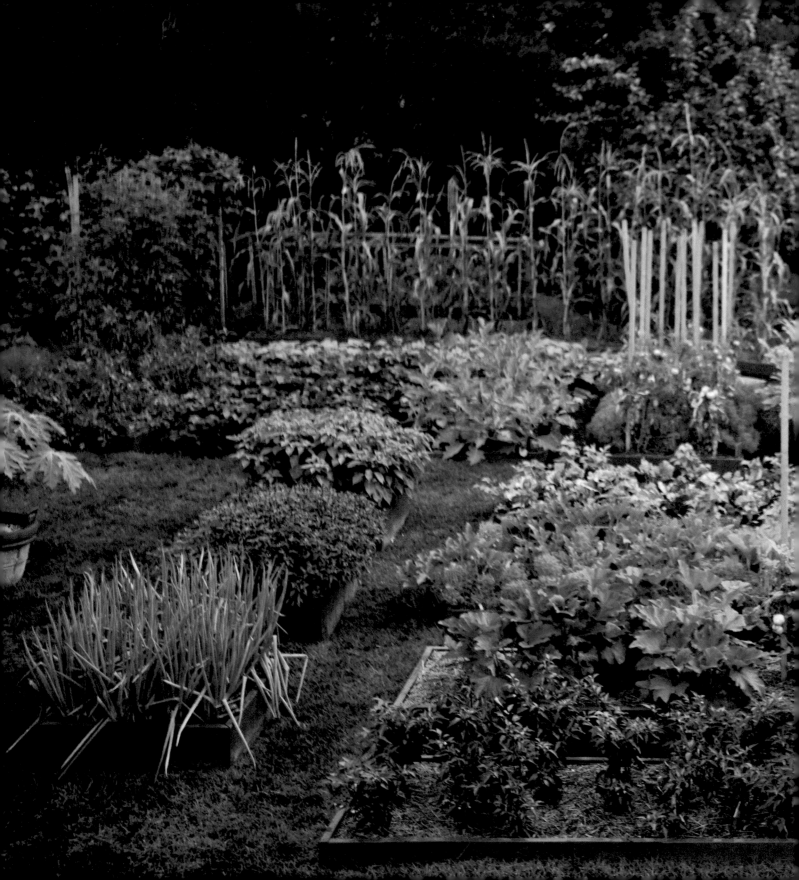

THE SUMMER GARDEN 2011

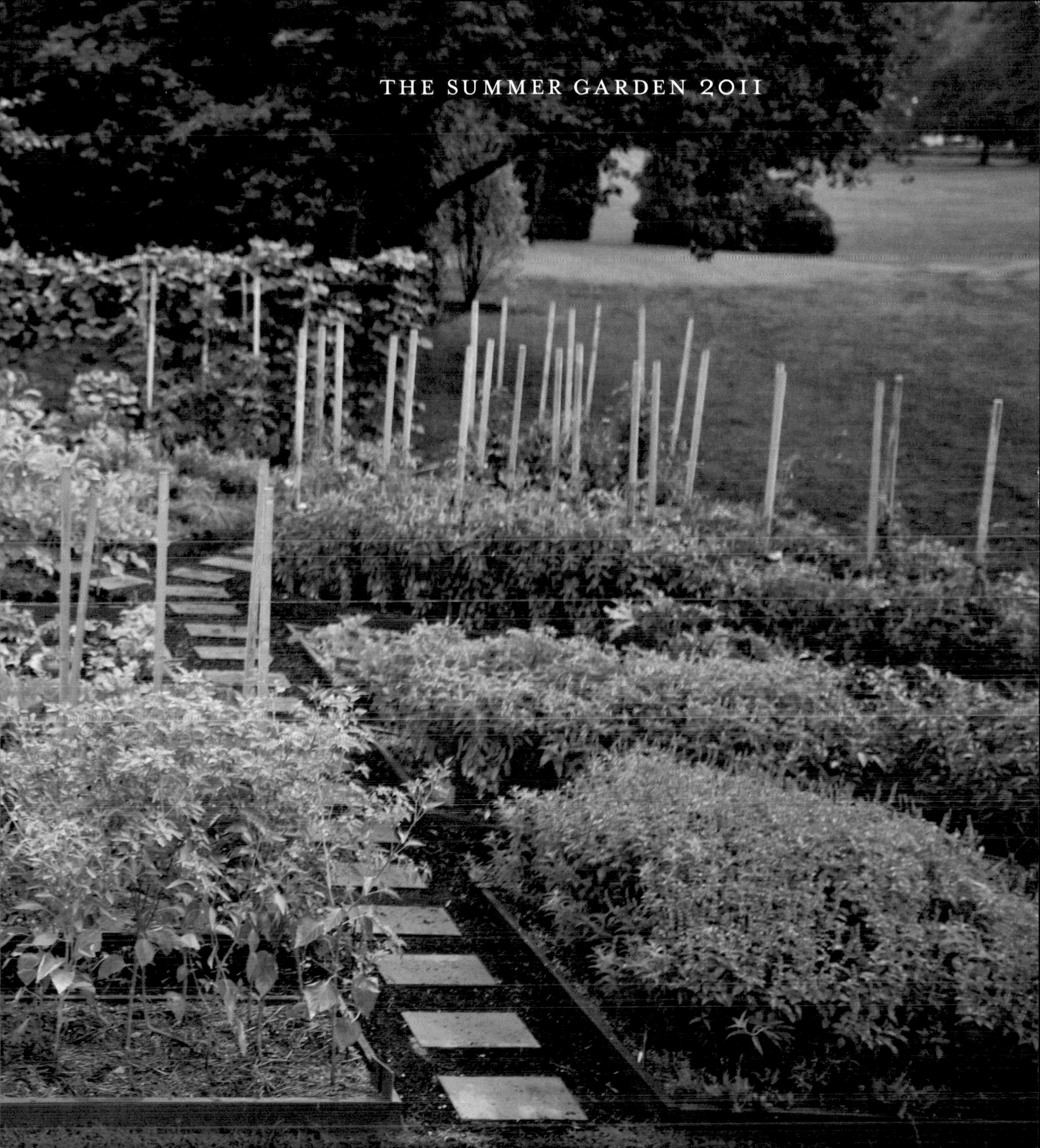

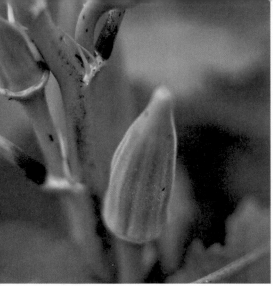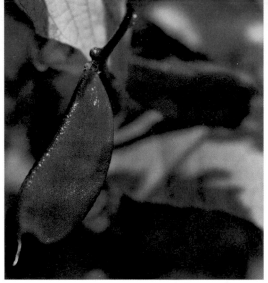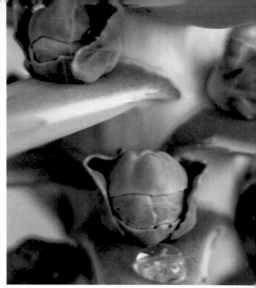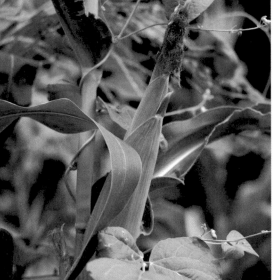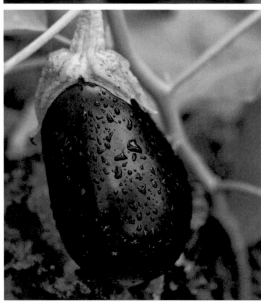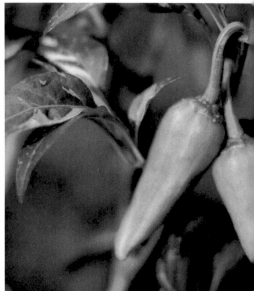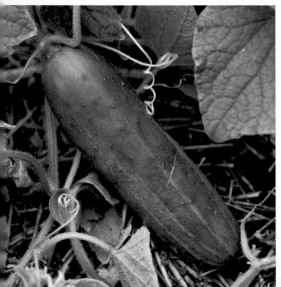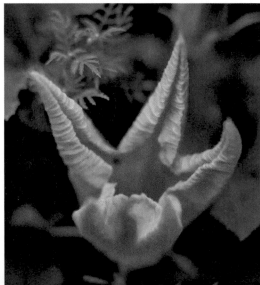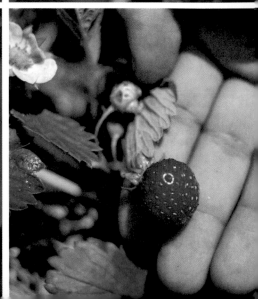

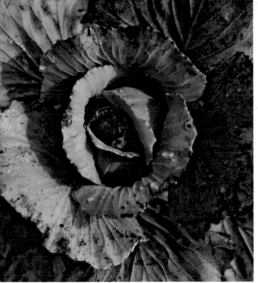 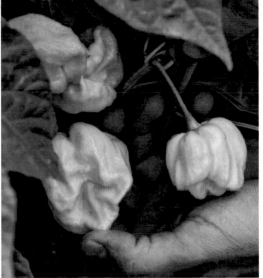 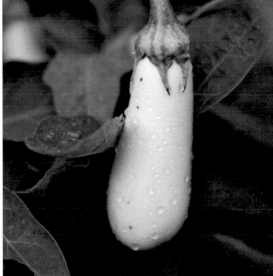

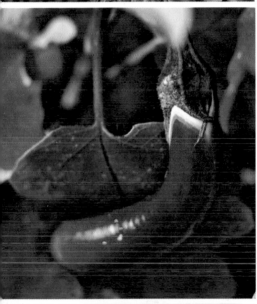 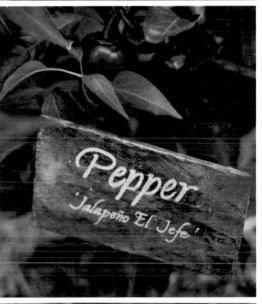 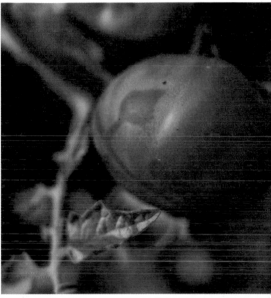

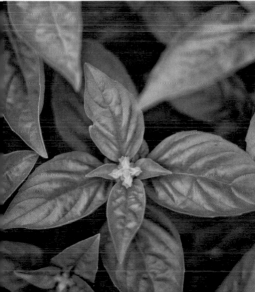 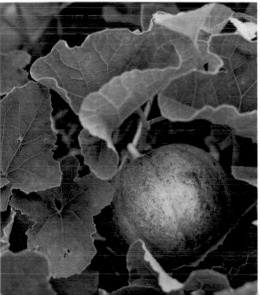 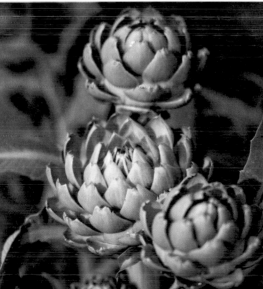

Pepper

'Jalapeño El Jefe'

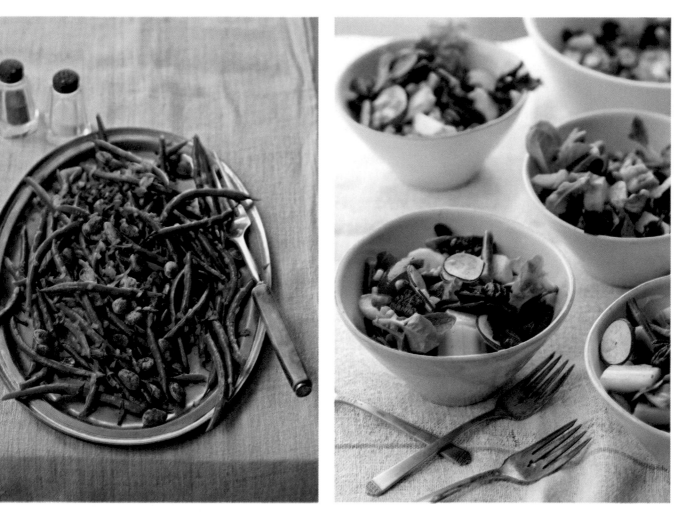

green beans with almonds
page 231

summer chopped salad
page 232

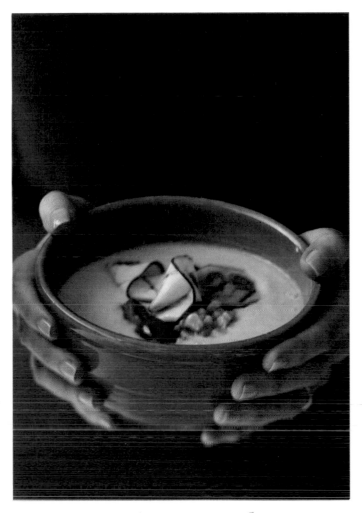

corn soup with
summer vegetables
page 234

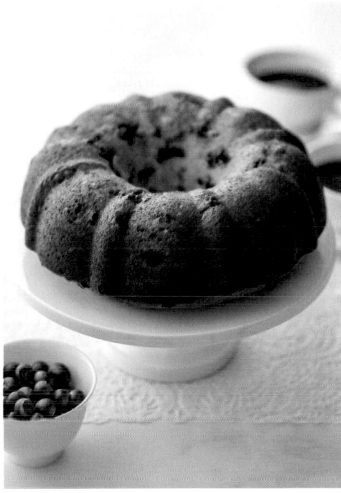

buttermilk blueberry
bundt cake
page 237

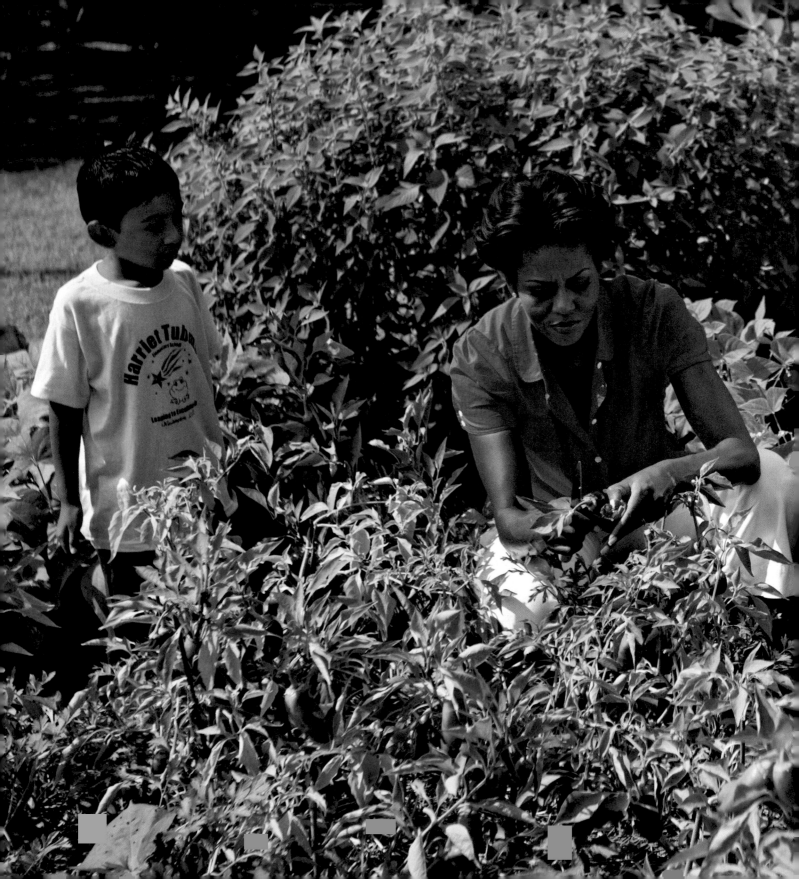

FINAL THOUGHTS ON SUMMER

Summer is a season of growth not just for our gardens but also for our communities. It's a time when we can come together, and work together, with our friends and neighbors, forming and strengthening friendships and discovering the many hopes, dreams, and aspirations that we share.

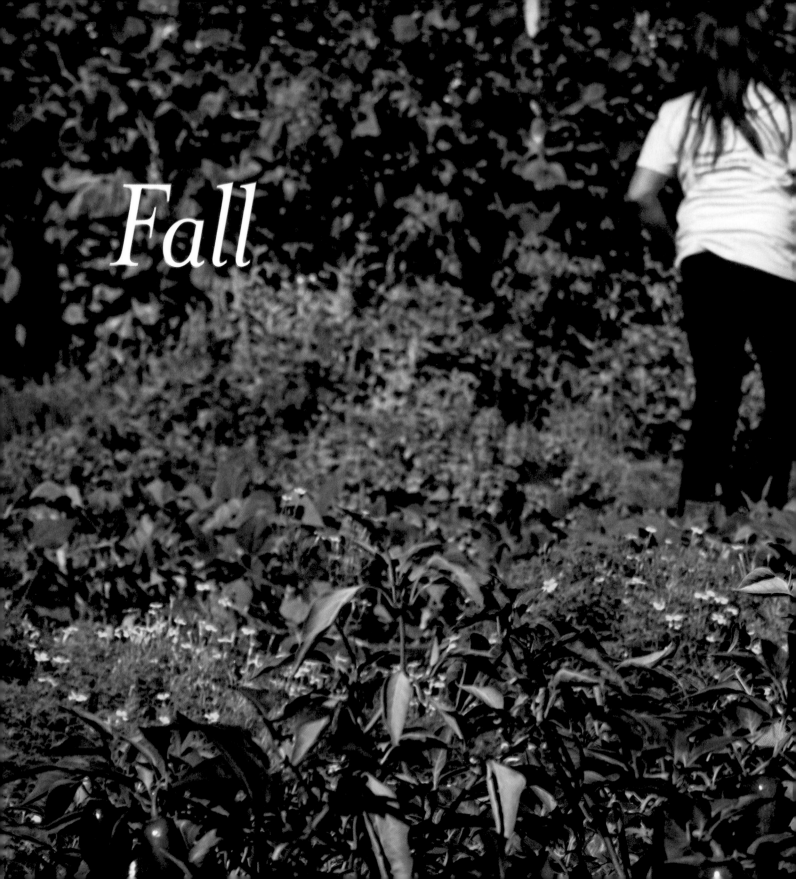

Fall

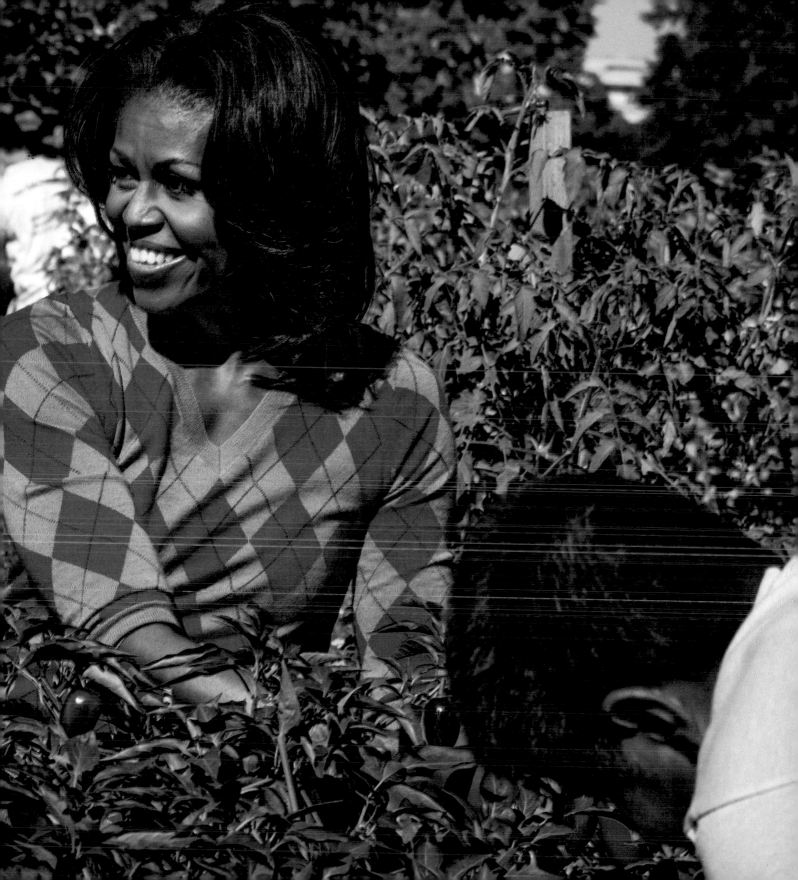

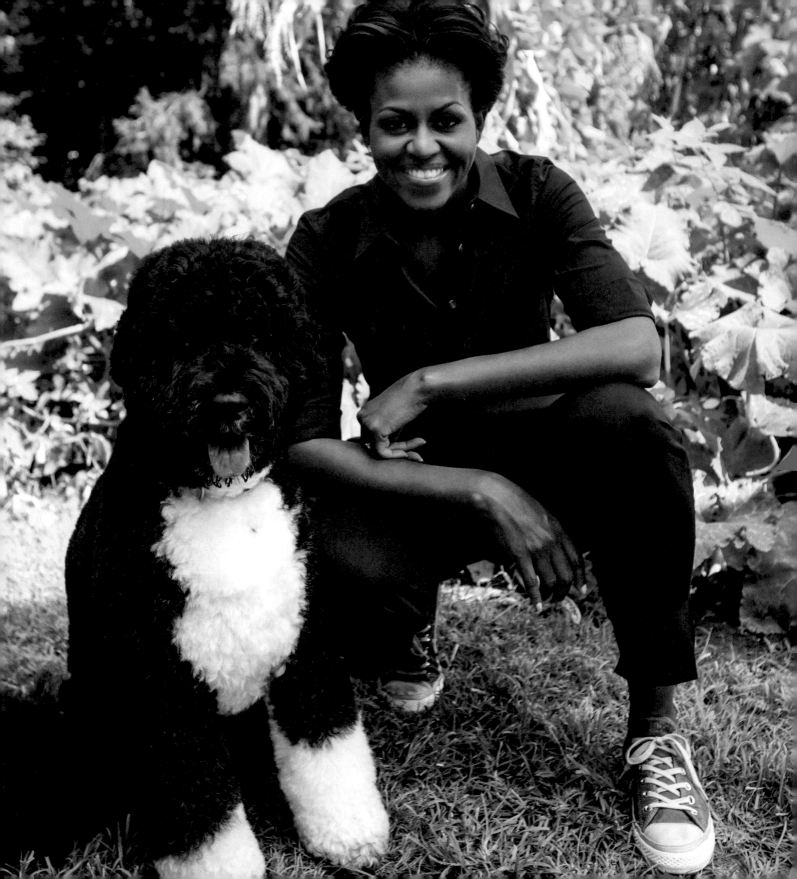

Fall: Harvesting and Sharing the Fruits (and Vegetables) of Our Labors

For us, fall is the main harvest season, a time when we reap the fruits (and vegetables) of all those months of hard work. But our gardens yield far more than fresh, delicious food. Individuals and organizations across our country are also using their harvests to help others by feeding the hungry, bringing fresh food into underserved neighborhoods, educating our children, and inspiring the next generation of gardeners.

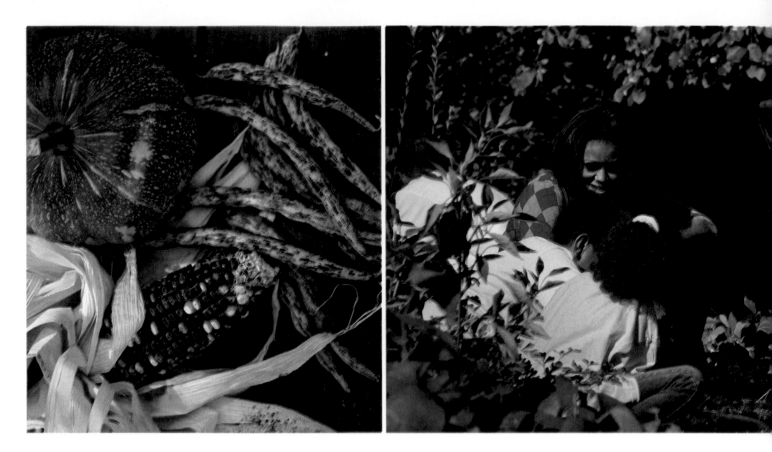

In the Kitchen Garden, harvest day often turns into a treasure hunt. Eager children—and grown-ups—can hardly wait to see what we have grown. Having watched the garden grow from that first planting to the final harvest, as some of our student volunteers have done, they have a sense of pride, ownership, and connection to the food they eat. On planting day, the kids learned how to sow seeds and how to squeeze down on the bottom of a cup to remove a delicate seedling. Months later, when the kids pull squash from the vines or twist off a ripe tomato or dig a sweet potato out of the ground, they see what those tiny seeds and seedlings have become.

Harvest day is a time of discovery. When a child pulls a root from the ground, at first it may not look like anything. But then, all of a sudden, when the dirt is brushed off, it's a vegetable they recognize—a sweet potato or a radish. For example, in 2009, we put in our first beds of sweet potatoes. When it came time to harvest them that fall, I gathered with children from Bancroft and Harriet Tubman elementary schools in Washington, and we

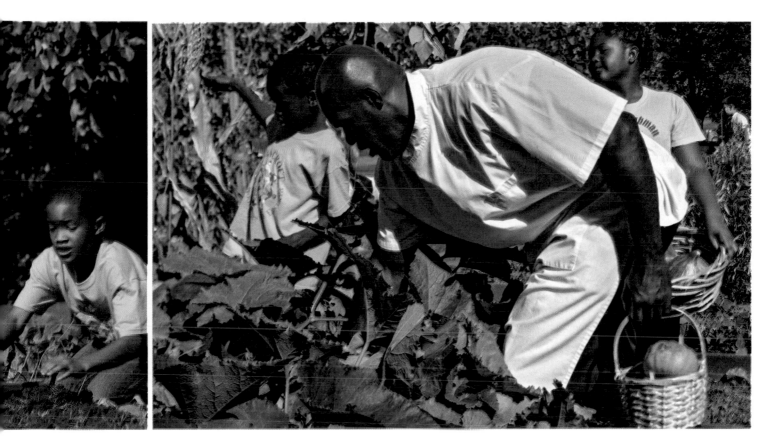

stood around what looked like a big scraggly bush. But when we cut away the jumble of vines and started digging, up from the ground came these massive sweet potatoes. I was shocked at how big they had grown! I watched the kids' faces glow and listened to their oohs and aahs. Before long, they were competing to see which of them could dig up the biggest sweet potato.

That level of enthusiasm is pretty typical. In fact, whenever we invite kids to help us harvest the garden, I'm struck by their eagerness, diligence, and focus. I'll never forget the day when we hosted preschool-age kids in the garden for the very first time. Two of the little girls were so excited to be part of the harvest that they didn't just pull the peppers off the plants; they pulled out the entire pepper plant. They didn't just pull off an herb stem; they pulled the whole herb out of the ground, roots and all. At first we tried to stop them, but those two were so focused and engaged that we just laughed and let them have at it. Someday I hope they'll look back and laugh at how they tried to make a clean sweep of the vegetable beds at the White House.

OUR 2011 FALL HARVEST
Everyone, kids and adults, is excited to have a full basket on harvest day.

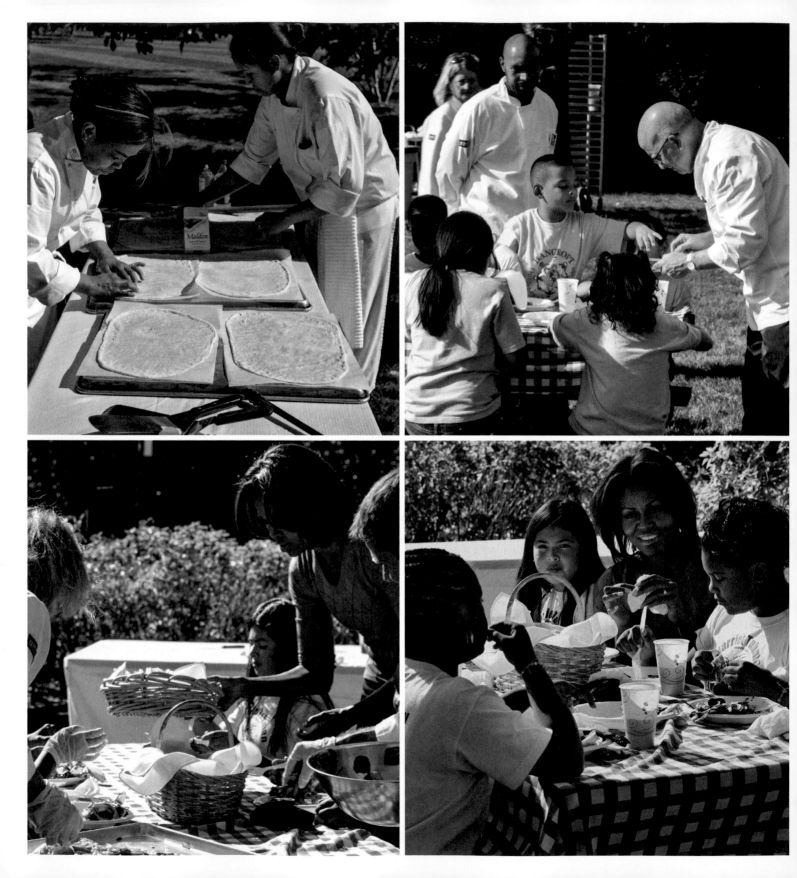

Tasting Our Harvest

As excited as kids are to harvest what they've planted, they're often even more excited to taste it. That's why cooking has always been an important part of our harvest tradition. Cooking and eating together is one of the best ways for kids and families to reap the benefits of growing their own food. And at the White House Kitchen Garden, we want kids to witness the entire journey of their food, from soil to table. So at our very first fall harvest, we invited them into the White House kitchen, where they helped cook a meal of grilled chicken, salad, brown rice, peas, and honey cupcakes. We didn't know whether the kids would like the vegetables, but they devoured the salad and asked for more.

In 2011, our chefs used ingredients from our harvest to cook a meal for a hungry crowd of student gardeners. They created pizza, made from grilled flatbread, cheese, and fresh garden vegetables (which our gardeners had picked and chopped themselves) roasted on portable, backyard grills. When the pizzas were served, at first some of the kids hesitated, staring uncertainly at their veggie-laden slices. But when they saw their friends starting to eat, they decided to give it a try.

Soon there wasn't much talking at the table, just a lot of contented chewing. The verdict was almost unanimous: Seconds, please. One child declared, "This is better than take-out pizza." Another said, "I want my mom to make this at home."

Several months later, I got a similar response from late-night host Jay Leno when I served him a slice of our veggie pizza on his show. An avowed vegetable-phobe, even he grudgingly admitted that it was "not bad."

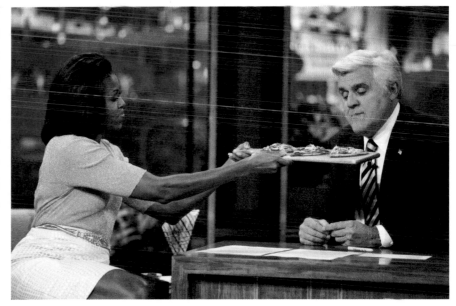

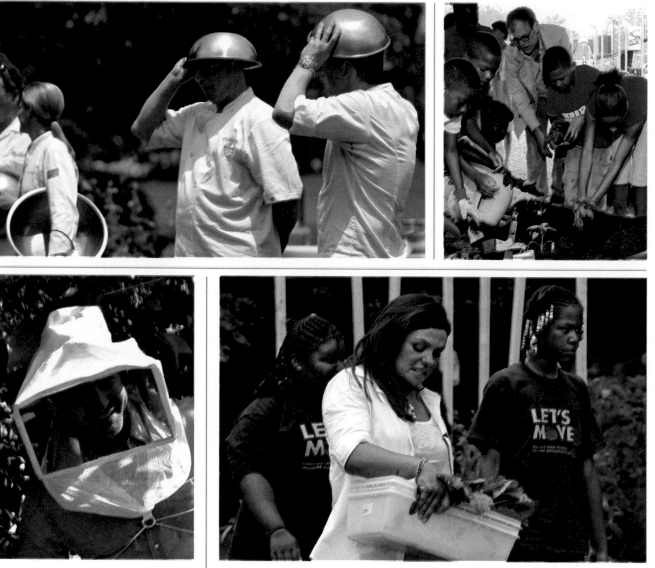

You don't have to be a kid to have fun in the garden. A number of famous chefs and other celebrities have come to the White House to help promote healthy eating and had a blast in the process. If the Kitchen Garden had a highlights reel, you'd see *Top Chef* head judge Tom Colicchio doing his best imitation of the eighties rock group Devo, covering his head with a metal salad bowl as he tried to deflect the sun's rays on a 90-plus-degree day in June. Or you'd catch TV design star Nate Berkus donning a mesh beekeeper's hat to get up close and personal with our beehive. *Iron Chef* host Alton Brown found himself flat on his back in the sweet potato bed when he decided to walk backward (unsuccessfully) through the garden. Rachael Ray had her own memorable moment. Whenever we invite guests to a harvest, we walk everyone out to the beds together to show them where they will be going and what they'll be doing. Rachael was assigned to the tomatoes, and when she saw them she couldn't wait. She began filling her basket before anyone else was ready to start. We teased Rachael that we were going to send her back to harvest school to learn to wait for the official group kickoff. And I'll never forget Heisman trophy winner and NFL quarterback Sam Bradford, whose MVP hands are usually wrapped around a football, delicately pulling peas off the vine and cutting lettuce.

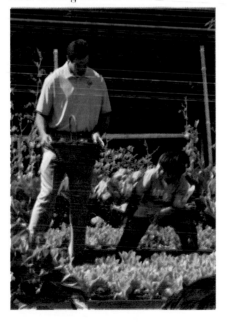

By 2010, we had two harvests under our belt, and we had enjoyed great success cooking with the kids. But we decided that this year we wanted to kick things up a notch by serving the food raw, fresh from the garden. I have to admit, we were a little worried that the kids would take one bite of a freshly rinsed veggie and really not like it—or that they wouldn't be willing to try it at all. As every parent knows, it can sometimes be hard to get kids to eat vegetables they're familiar with, let alone to try new ones.

The moment of truth arrived when we set out the platters of fresh broccoli, spinach, peas, and cauliflower. The kids gathered around, as did the press—about fifty reporters watching every move. At that moment, one ten-year-old girl approached the table and took not just one piece of raw cauliflower, not just a handful of it—she actually picked up the whole platter and carried it over to the picnic benches, where she sat down and started stuffing the florets into her mouth until her cheeks bulged.

Sam Kass approached her, worried that something was wrong. But she looked up at him, beaming with pride, and said with her mouth full, "This is so great. What is it?" Sam jokes that it is the first time he ever had to ask a child to stop eating her vegetables (we wanted everyone to get a taste). After planting these vegetables, watching them grow, and harvesting them, this girl was open to—and excited about—trying them. When she did, she realized that they tasted good. That is the power of a single garden, a single fresh vegetable, to expand the horizons of our young people.

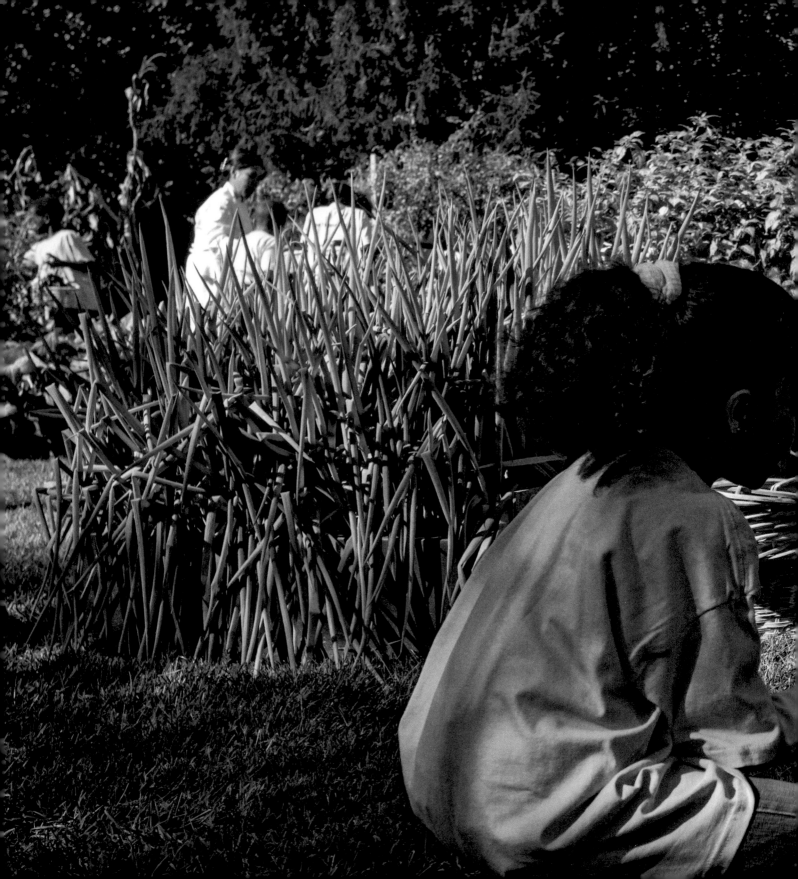

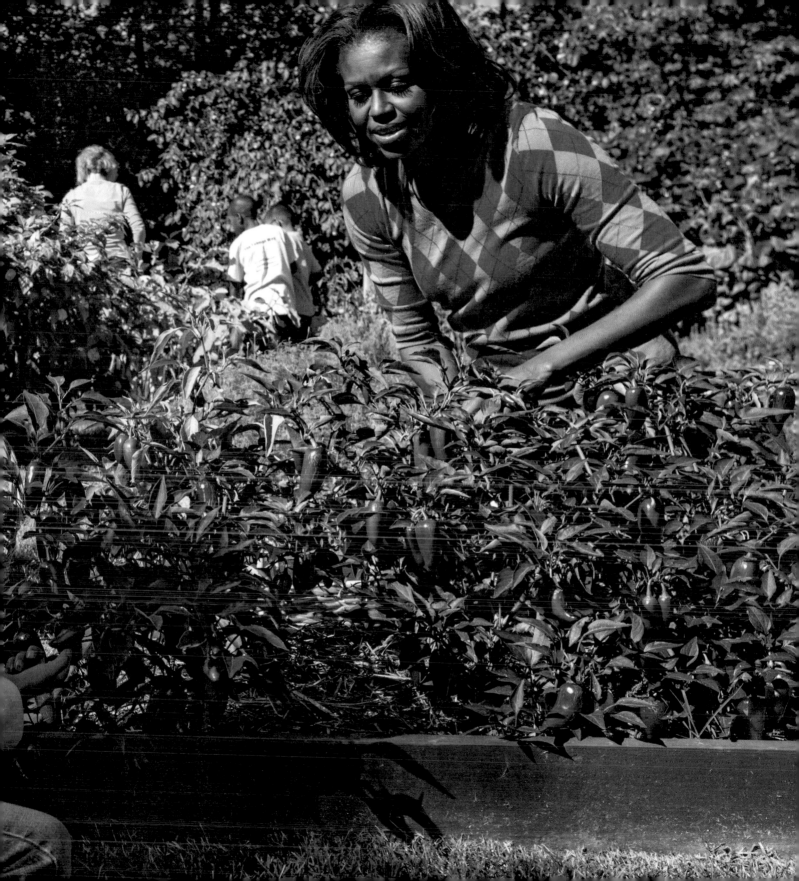

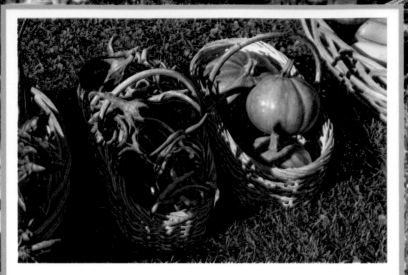

THE HUNT FOR THE PERFECT PUMPKIN: AN IMPORTANT HARVEST LESSON

In the White House Kitchen Garden, we learned early on that despite our best efforts, we can't always predict what we'll harvest. When we started the garden, we knew we wanted to grow pumpkins, and we hoped for big ones that the kids could harvest and Malia and Sasha could carve as jack-o'-lanterns for Halloween. In 2009, we planted our seeds and eagerly watched and waited, and watched and waited, and after months and months we had vines but no pumpkins. It turned out that the summer was too hot, and we had planted our pumpkin seeds too late.

The second year, we planted the pumpkins sooner, but it was still not quite soon enough; by midsummer, it looked like there would be no pumpkins again. The garden team debated ripping out the vines, but in one last-ditch effort, they got down on their knees and pollinated the pumpkin blossoms by hand. After all that work, all we got was one orange pumpkin and four semi-orange pumpkins. But we were so proud of that single orange pumpkin! It made the rounds of the White House offices for weeks before it was eventually carved.

In 2011, despite planting our pumpkin seeds earlier, we once again came up empty on pumpkins. But we had a bumper crop of Seminole squash from our Three Sisters planting, enough to make a delicious squash soup for the Republic of Korea State Dinner. And now I'm wondering, is it possible to carve a Seminole squash and start a new tradition?

How Our Gardens Can Help Those in Need

My husband and I have both been tremendously blessed in our lives. Barack was raised by his grandparents and by a single mother who struggled to pay the bills, and neither of my parents attended college. But they all saved and sacrificed so that we could get an education and have opportunities they never dreamed of. So we both feel an obligation—personally and professionally—to give something back and lift up others the way our families lifted us. From the beginning, I wanted the garden to be part of that work, but I wasn't exactly sure how. During one of the first service projects I participated in after moving to Washington—serving lunch at Miriam's Kitchen, an organization that helps homeless individuals in the D.C. area—I found my answer.

Miriam's Kitchen is located in a church basement just eight blocks from the White House, and every week they prepare more than one thousand healthy breakfasts and dinners, all for $1 or less per meal.

We came to Miriam's at the invitation of Steve Badt, the Executive Chef, and the moment I arrived, he put me to work. My job was to dish out the mushroom risotto, accompanied by steamed broccoli, homemade apple-carrot muffins, wheat rolls, and salad. The staff and volunteers take great

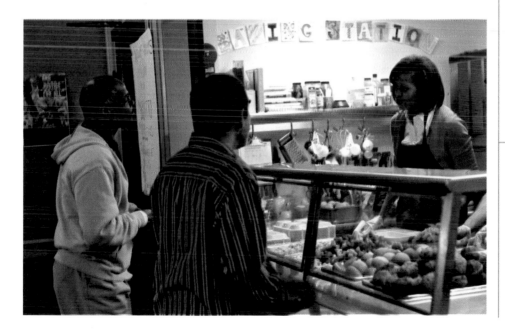

SERVING OTHERS
One of my first service projects in Washington, D.C., was serving lunch to the guests at Miriam's Kitchen, which prides itself on offering healthy, fresh, delicious food to those in need.

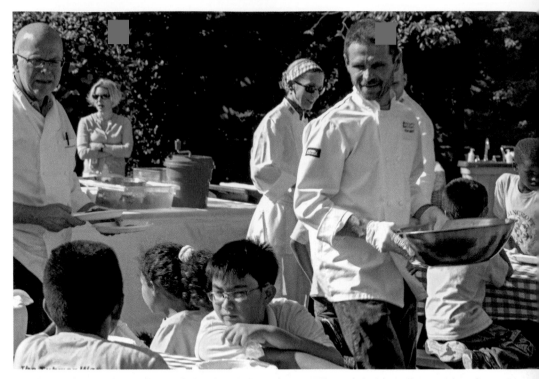

SHARING OUR HARVEST
Steve Badt, Executive Chef for Miriam's Kitchen, joins us at our Fall 2011 Harvest.

pride in the high quality of the food they serve. Their philosophy is that if someone comes there and will get only one meal, it should be the very best meal they can have. They see each of the more than four thousand people who pass through their doors each year as guests, and they want their guests to get the same level of nutrition and pleasure in their food as those of us who are more fortunate.

We invited Steve to join us to help pick vegetables at our first fall harvest in the White House Kitchen Garden, and afterward we donated some of that produce to Miriam's Kitchen. Every year since then, throughout the growing season, we've sent over hand-packed boxes of our vegetables, donating roughly a third of all the produce we grow. Sharing our harvest like this is one of the highlights of each season.

But difficulties accessing—and affording—fresh, healthy food aren't limited to those struggling with serious hardship. Today, millions of American families are living in so-called food deserts, communities without a single grocery store and no convenient access to fresh, nutritious food. So if parents want to buy some fruit for their children's lunches, or a head of lettuce for a salad at dinner, they may need to take two or three city buses or pay a fortune for a taxi to another community. As a result, many families end up buying their groceries at local gas station mini-marts or convenience stores—places that offer few, if any, healthy options—and many children don't get the basic nutrition they need to grow up healthy.

This is unacceptable. In this country, no matter where we live, we should all be able to provide nutritious food for our families. And today, many communities rely on gardens to make that aspiration a reality. In cities and towns across America, people are coming together, pooling their time, energy, and resources, and growing their own fresh, nutritious, and affordable food. The Camden City Garden Club in Camden, New Jersey, is one example of this kind of effort.

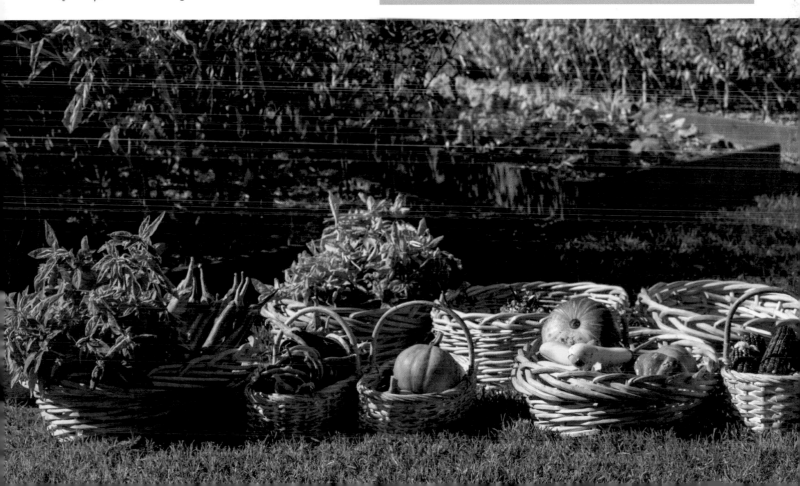

Camden City Garden Club, CAMDEN, NEW JERSEY

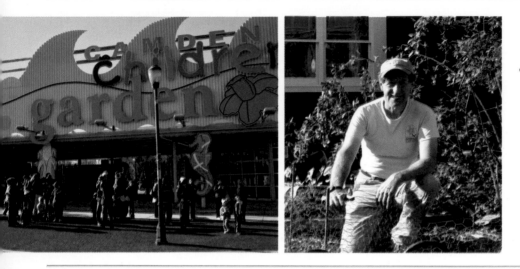

"Our gardeners put a lot of heart and soul and sweat equity into their plots."

—MIKE DEVLIN,
President, Camden City Garden Club

Camden was recently listed as one of the nine most underserved, food-insecure communities in America. But according to a University of Pennsylvania study, Camden also has the fastest-growing community gardening program in the nation. Over the past four years, the number of gardens assisted by the Camden City Garden Club has risen from fewer than 40 to more than 116, and they have a waiting list of 30 more.

"**Y**ou have to leave the city to go buy healthy food, and our residents spend a lot of their income just to purchase food. When the last economic downturn hit, the interest in community gardening exploded. And there are thousands of abandoned lots, many of which could be used to grow fresh produce. Now the city of Camden is allowing people to adopt lots. We're just beginning to keep up with the demand.

"I had an English grandmother who taught me how to garden. For years, when I worked as a lawyer and was in politics, I escaped them both by going into the garden. Then, in 1985, my wife, Valerie Frick, and I started the Camden Community Gardening Program. At first it was just meant to be a way to expand community gardening. But our city needed so much more than that. We started the Camden Children's Garden, a youth employment and training program, a school education program, and we also help community gardeners maintain well over one hundred sites. Each year, we give out about two hundred thousand plants. Some plants are raised by our youth program, we buy some, some are donated from nurseries, and we also get last year's leftover seeds donated by a seed company.

"When we started the club, most of the people interested in growing were predominantly older folks, many African Americans who had grown up in the South and had migrated here. Many had a farming background. Now we're getting a lot of younger people, many from South America and Southeast Asia. Some have never planted anything before. Eighty to one hundred people attend our monthly meetings. We've turned the meetings into healthy food events and nutrition/gardening workshops. We pick seasonable vegetables and grill them. One month it was asparagus. Most people had never tried it, but they got to taste it and really liked it. When it's harvest time, we have

'Ground to Grill BBQs,' healthy barbecues for 150 community gardeners and their children.

"Here gardeners pick up the spirit of gardening and run with it. They start growing on a lot and then they start cleaning up the lots around them. We have thirty churches and thirty-four community organizations that have started community gardens with us, as well as eighty-five backyard gardeners. We also have gardens tucked away in empty spaces along a creek that runs through the city.

"We're one of the poorest cities, and the second-most-dangerous city in the nation, but 100 percent of our gardeners grow surplus crops and give them away. Our gardeners grow more than five hundred thousand pounds of fresh food a year on twenty-five acres, and according to the University of Pennsylvania, about 10 percent of Camden's population gets some of their produce from our programs."

—MIKE DEVLIN

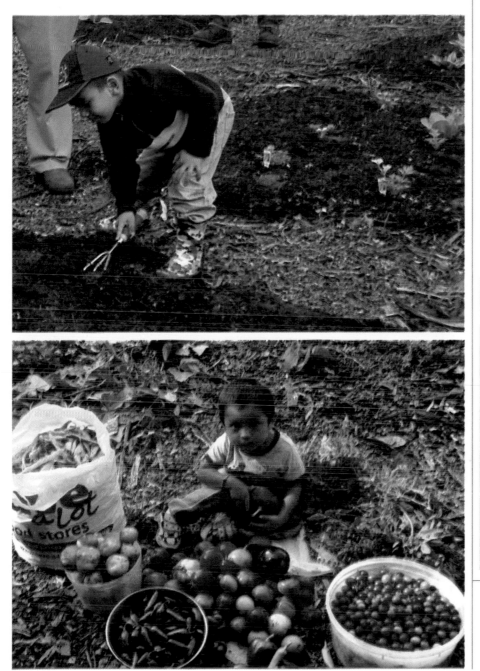

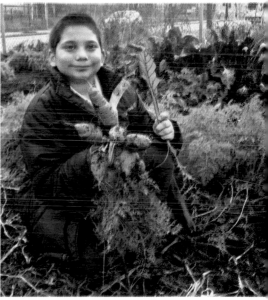

TRANSFORMING A CITY
The Camden City Garden Club is lifting up a struggling city, one plant and one garden at a time.

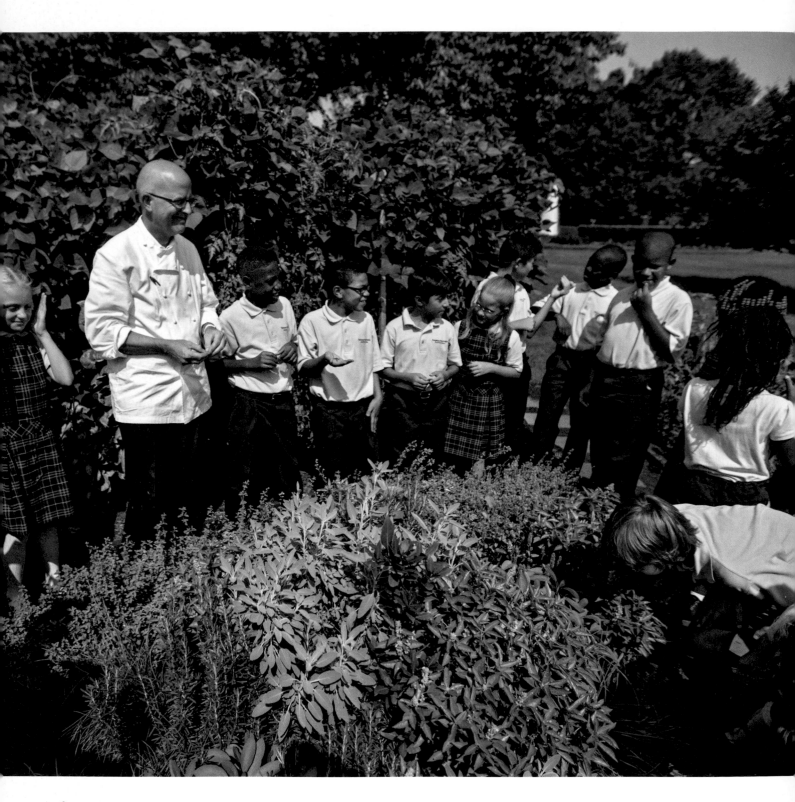

How Our Gardens Can Educate and Inspire Our Children

Gardens can be used not just to nourish our children's bodies but to nourish their minds and shape their habits and preferences as well. When we engage children in harvesting our gardens—when we teach them about where their food comes from, how to prepare it, and how to grow it themselves—they reap the benefits well into the future. These early lessons about nutrition can affect the choices they make about what they eat for the rest of their lives—and that can determine what they feed their own children decades from now. For many young people, school gardens and youth gardening programs across this country have been the starting point for this journey.

Here are a few of their stories.

A BRIEF HISTORY OF SCHOOL GARDENS

We are not the first generation to plant school gardens. The first official school garden in the United States was actually planted in Roxbury, Massachusetts, in 1891; the students grew flowers and vegetables. As America became more urbanized, school gardens were incorporated into nature study programs. Within fifteen years, there were more than seventy-five thousand school gardens across the country. During World War I, a popular motto was, "A garden for every child. Every child in a garden." School gardening was also widespread throughout World War II, when victory gardens were frequently grown on school grounds. But by the 1950s, the garden had largely disappeared from the educational landscape.

Today school gardens are making a comeback. Whether it's a few containers in a sunny corner of a concrete school yard or a large square of cultivated land beside school playing fields, school gardens have become outdoor classrooms, teaching everything from science and ecology to history and culture to nutrition. For many students, these gardens are their only chance to learn about where their food actually comes from.

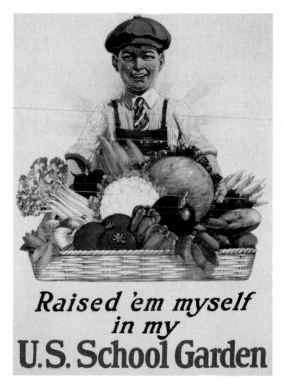

Raised 'em myself in my U.S. School Garden

How Two Brooklyn Schools Made Empty Spaces Bloom

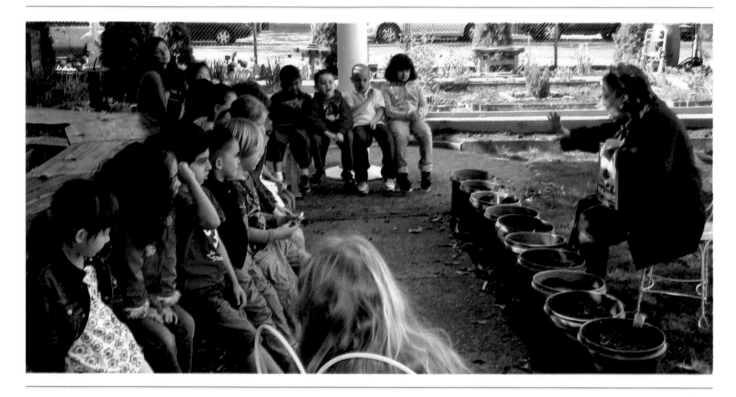

PS 102: The lot-size yard next to this elementary school, which once housed a World War II victory garden, was nothing but unused space. At one point it was little more than a catchall for trash. Now it is a garden that has grown everything from pumpkins to cacti. Because PS 102's soil isn't viable for gardening, the school relies on a container garden system, a vertical gardening system (allowing plants to grow from floor to ceiling along a wall), and sub-irrigated planters (planters in which water is introduced at the roots of the plants, soaking upward). The planters were donated by a neighbor and garden supporter across the street, and the clean soil they provide allows the school to serve some of what it grows in the lunchroom.

"We've been trying to do as much as we can with the space," Margaret Sheri, parent coordinator at PS 102, explains. That includes a butterfly garden and an annual Arbor Day Read Aloud. In addition, because PS 102 has three classes of visually impaired students, one parent came up with the idea of planting a "scratch-and-sniff garden," with soft leaves to touch and fragrant herbs—such as fennel, lemon balm, sage, and oregano—to smell.

Much of the garden is maintained by the parents. "I have parents who want to work twenty hours in the mud, and parents who want to bake cookies and run the open-house table. We have space for everyone and a great group of volunteers. What I've learned is that if you build it, they will come," adds Sheri.

There are a few residents in the neighborhood who remember the original World War II victory garden that once stood on that spot. For some, those early memories led to a lifelong love of gardening. The parents, teachers, and volunteers at PS 102 hope that their garden will have a similar impact on the school's students today.

A TEACHING GARDEN
Students at PS 102 enjoy an Arbor Day Read Aloud in the garden. Caring for the garden has also led the kids to care for the neighborhood.

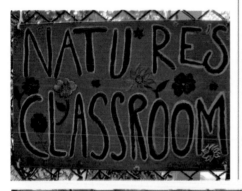

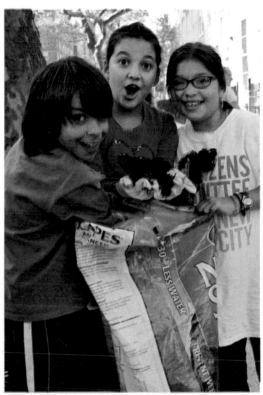

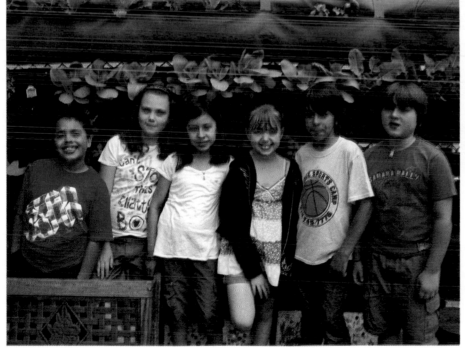

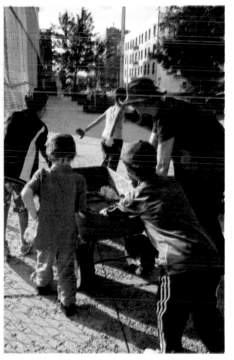

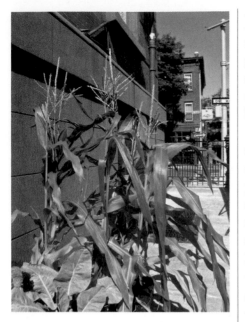

CORN GROWS IN BROOKLYN

"We are an urban school, with no field in back, in the middle of brownstone Brooklyn. Now our kids know food doesn't just come from the bodega on the corner."
—Mary Vines

PS 107: There wasn't a single tree or blade of grass on the school grounds at PS 107, and the only open space was a north-facing concrete courtyard, surrounded on three sides by the school building.

But over the course of five years, a group of parents set up nineteen container systems, several half-barrel planters, and a donated nine-foot self-watering planter alongside six raised beds, which were built by a neighborhood carpenter who donated his time. The space has been named the Sunshine Garden, and here students have raised an impressive variety of vegetables and herbs.

They've faced plenty of challenges, from lack of sunlight to working around scaffolding for building repairs, to pests ranging from hungry birds (who ate the cucumbers) to cabbage butterflies (who attacked the kale

and broccoli). Then, in the fall of 2010, just after the scaffolding came down and the school was preparing for its big harvest, a tornado and hailstorm swept through the area, destroying most of the crops. "It was a humbling experience for the gardeners, who lost their harvest just as a farmer would to a sudden storm," says PS 107 parent Michele Israel. But the garden was replanted and flourished once again the next spring.

Today the school gardeners are using seasonal gardening techniques and timing their planting to extend the growing and harvest seasons to line up with the beginning and end of the school year. Teachers have begun incorporating the garden into their lesson plans, educating students about the nutritional value of fruits and vegetables and helping them study the effects of the weather

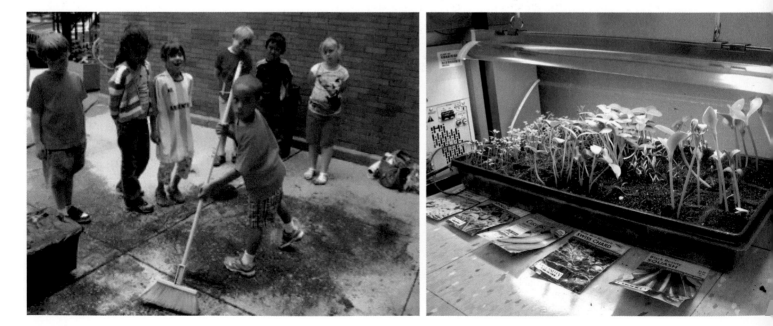

on their plants. One teacher even organized a Three Sisters planting as a way for students to learn about Native American cultures and traditions. The garden has also spurred the school to change the lunch menu to include more healthy offerings and a salad bar.

"The garden was a wish for many, many years," says PTA president Mary Vines. "Most of our kids don't have their own outdoor space. Now they have a place where they can plant a seed and watch it grow—they feel it, touch it, and smell it. They can see the miracle of life, and we can say to them, 'This is your space and your garden.'"

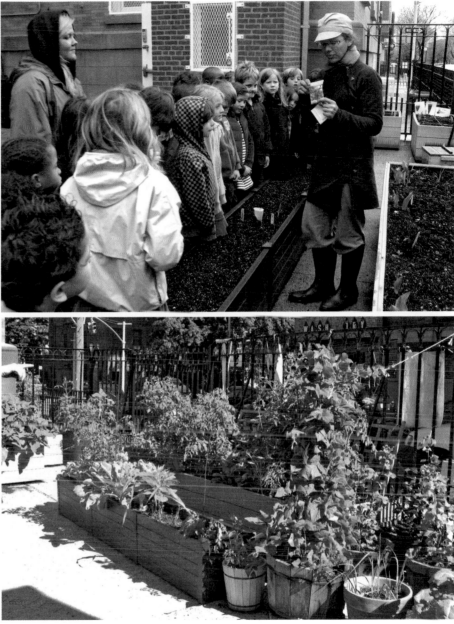

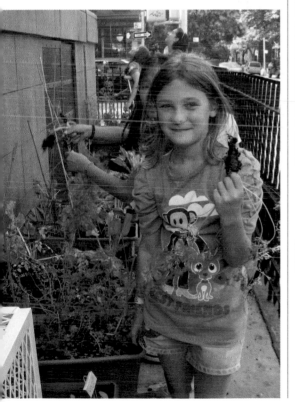

FROM SPRING PLANTING TO FULL BOUNTY

"Kids feel a great sense of ownership, 'that's my plant.' My son grew a green bean and then he got to eat it. He would have never eaten it if I had given it to him." —Mary Vines

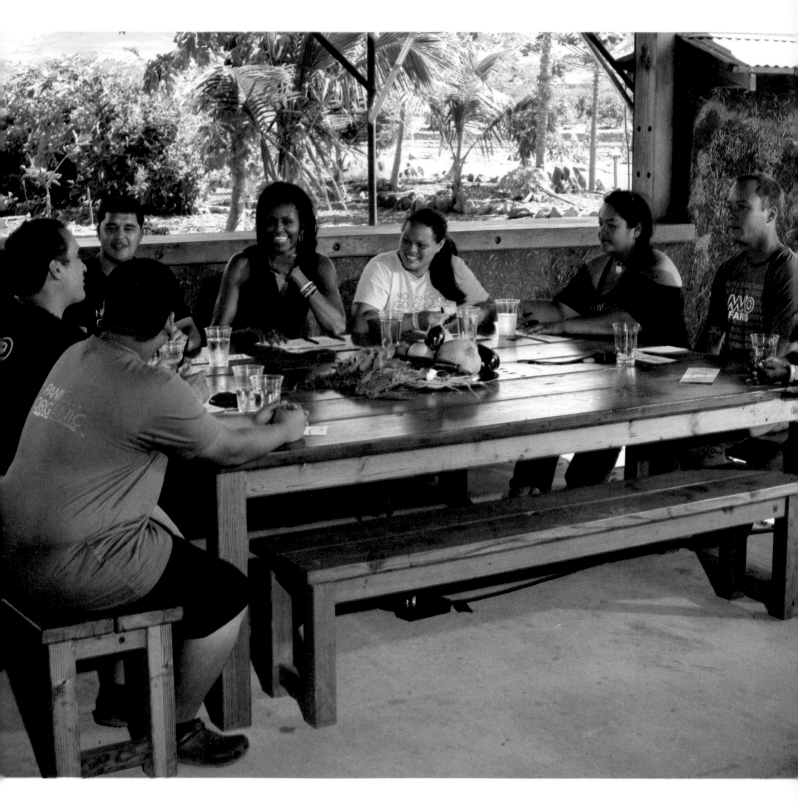

A GARDEN EDUCATION FOR KIDS AND THEIR COMMUNITY

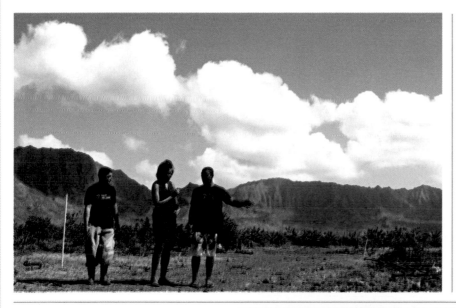

GROWING A BETTER FUTURE
The MA'O Organic Farms in Waianae on the island of Oahu is reconnecting many local young people with Hawaiian traditions. During my visit, they shared their stories and their dreams with me.

In November 2011, I had the privilege of visiting MA'O Organic Farms on the Hawaiian Island of Oahu. MA'O is committed to helping one of the poorest communities in Hawaii return to its roots of farming and native planting. They grow thirty-five different fruits and vegetables on their twenty-four acres, and the farmers at MA'O are primarily young people who spend twenty hours a week working on the farm in exchange for tuition waivers at a local college and a monthly stipend (which is often the primary support for their families). Some of these farmer-apprentices told me that as a result of what they've learned on the farm, they have

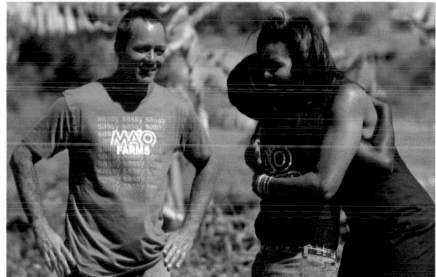

changed their own diets and are working to share their knowledge about healthy eating with their families and community. "It's bigger than just going to school," farmer and student Maisha Abbott told me. "It's about changing our community."

Growing Power, MILWAUKEE, WISCONSIN

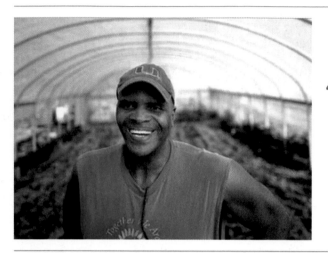

"Our motto is simple: to grow food, to grow minds, and to grow community."

—WILL ALLEN,
Founder, Growing Power

Urban farmer Will Allen of Milwaukee, Wisconsin, came to the White House in February 2010 to help me launch Let's Move! *Will's story reminds us that gardens are educating and inspiring children not just in schools but in places ranging from farms to churches to afterschool programs. Through his work with Growing Power, Will shows us how gardens can transform young people's lives.*

"I grew up in Rockville, Maryland, where my parents had a small farm. My father and mother moved to the Washington, D.C., area in the 1930s; both had been sharecroppers. Most people who moved north wanted to leave farming, but not my parents. My mother did domestic work and my father was a construction laborer, but they always rented a plot to farm. They raised vegetables and chickens and gave most of the excess food away to extended family and friends.

People would show up at our house around six every night to eat at my mother's table, and I got up early every morning to help them with the farm chores.

"In high school, I was an all-American basketball player and the first African American player to play at the University of Miami. When I left for college, I said that I was never going to do this hard farming work again. After college, I played a little pro ball and then went and played in the European leagues. When I moved back to the United States, I settled in Wisconsin, outside of Milwaukee, with my wife. I shared a couple of acres of farmland and worked up to buying one hundred acres from my wife's family. I farmed, and I worked as a district manager for a food service company and then in corporate marketing for Procter & Gamble. In 1993, I was driving around looking

for a place to sell my farm produce. I saw a For Sale sign on a lot with a bunch of A-frame greenhouses. It was a place called Growing Power, and it was a flower shop going out of business. I saw my future. With the greenhouses, I could grow indoors during the Milwaukee winters, and with the space, I could start working with kids and teaching them how to grow food and where food comes from.

"Today Growing Power is a multi-generational and multicultural program with twenty farms and seventy programs. We grow food year-round and train more than a thousand farmers each year. We have sixteen regional training centers across the United States. We have young people coming from colleges, rural communities, urban areas, and small towns. In addition to our two acres in the city of Milwaukee, we have four farms in Chicago, and we're build-

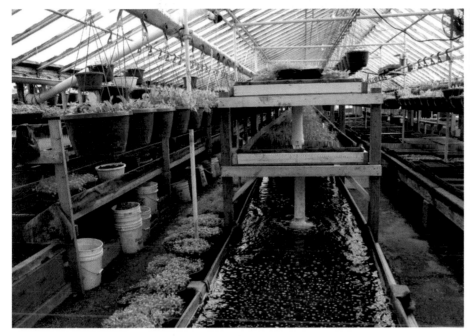

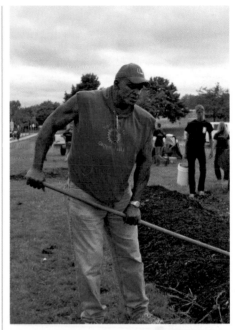

ing an agricultural charter school in an underserved section of Madison, Wisconsin. We have a worm farm that raises five thousand pounds of worms a year. We produce one hundred thousand pounds of compost. And we can feed ten thousand people a year out of our national headquarters in Milwaukee. Among other things, we provide a weekly market bag of fresh produce to low-income residents at a reduced cost.

"In Milwaukee, we're less than half a mile from the city's largest housing project, but it's more than three miles to the nearest Pick 'n Save. That's a long way if you have to carry your bags. Take-out food joints are a lot closer. People who live in underserved communities have a far higher incidence of diet-related health problems, like diabetes, heart disease, and obesity.

"But inside Growing Power's two acres, we have beets, chard, spinach, chickens, ducks, heritage turkeys, and beehives. We're even raising fresh fish with aquaponics, a sustainable food production system that combines raising aquatic animals such as fish in tanks with hydroponics (cultivating plants in water).

"In the city, when people ask for help, we try to be there. We've started gardens to grow crops at firehouses that have extra land. We have a twenty-year lease on land with the Milwaukee public school system to put in gardens. Things like this will have a huge impact. It's just going to take time. It takes about five years to learn how to become a beginning farmer. You have to learn everything from how to seed different crops to the amount of seed to use. At Growing Power, we've figured out how to use the heat from making compost

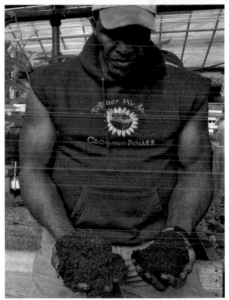

THE POWER OF GROWING

In addition to growing fruits and vegetables, Growing Power also raises fish in tanks (top, left). Good soil is one of the key building blocks of a healthy food system. Above, Will Allen holds his home-grown soil.

to keep our hoop houses (the greenhouses where we grow some of our crops) warm in the winter.

"I call all this the 'Good Food Revolution,' and it's got room to grow. There are thirty-three square miles of vacant land in Chicago, some seventy-seven thousand vacant lots, many of which could have gardens. We can't wait for major grocery stores to come into each community; we need to transition corner stores into getting better food. People in those communities know what good food is, they just need better access. Ninety-nine percent of the food sold in Milwaukee, Wisconsin, and Cleveland, Ohio, comes from outside of the region. If 10 percent of Milwaukee's food or Cleveland's food could be raised locally, that would be a $1 billion change to the local economy. We can provide high-quality, safe, healthy, and affordable food for all residents of our communities. And this can transform every level of a community. But we cannot have healthy communities without a healthy food system."

—WILL ALLEN

THE POWER OF GROWING POWER: CHICAGO

In October 2011, I had the chance to see Growing Power in action when I stopped by Will Allen's Iron Street Urban Farm on Chicago's South Side. Iron Street took over an old truck depot and turned its seven-acre building site into an oasis of urban agriculture. Now Will is raising both crops and "farm kids" in the middle of the city, and he does so with tremendous passion and imagination. I saw straw "chandelier" baskets that were being used to grow mushrooms from the ceiling, and I visited a workshop in the building where kids learn to repair bikes so they can deliver the freshly grown produce around the neighborhood. I also had the privilege of meeting some of these young men and women when a few of them treated me to an in-depth explanation of how to create the best compost—and I even made the acquaintance of a wriggling worm from that compost.

One of these students was a young man from a troubled background. When he first started working at Iron Street, he didn't say a word to anyone; he simply came to the farm each day and did whatever job the staff provided for him. But they welcomed him and encouraged him, and finally, after about two years of silence, he began to open up. He had been at the farm for eight years by the time I visited, and he proudly told me about all he had learned there.

Growing Power has taken the concept of "growing" to the next level, providing students with job training and opportunities for entrepreneurship. They're also hosting cooking demonstrations and opening farmers' markets in underserved communities. It is my hope that programs like Iron Street will open in communities across the country, providing opportunities like these to as many of our young people as possible.

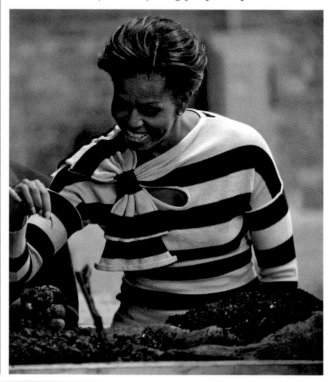

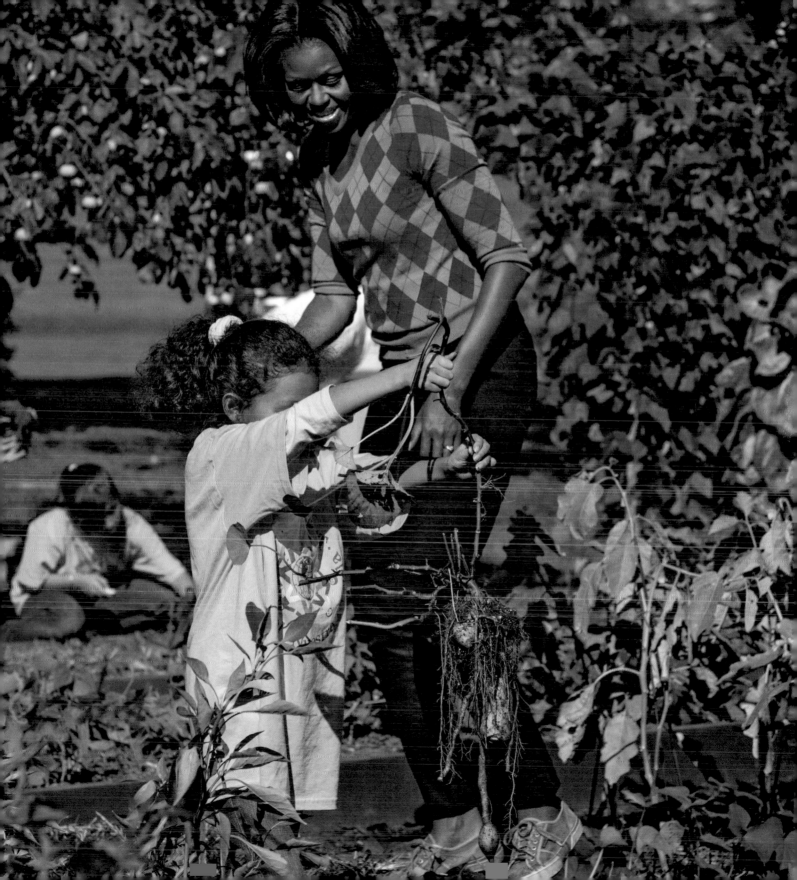

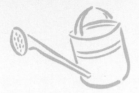

Engaging Our Children in Our Gardens: How to Build a Children's Garden
Thoughts from Jim Adams, National Park Service Supervisory Horticulturist

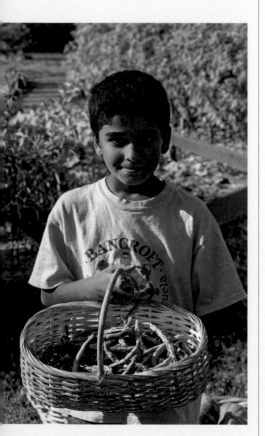

Growing a children's garden—a garden planted and harvested by, and for, children—is a great way to get kids involved in, and excited about, gardening.

Designing the Garden

ENGAGE THEIR SENSES

- Start with groupings of herbs, from basil to lemon verbena, which can highlight smell.
- Use plants of varying sizes with different textures, which can entice children to touch. Children notice the difference between the thin vine of a pea and the slightly wavy shell of a snow pea pod or between the fragile skin of a tomato and the thicker skin of an eggplant.

MAKE IT EXCITING

- Flowers, especially dramatic ones like sunflowers, are a great addition. Although they take up a lot of room, sunflowers can grow from a single seed to a two-foot-tall plant in a month, and they produce edible seeds that children can taste for themselves.

MAKE IT ACCESSIBLE

- Create clearly designed paths to allow children to walk through the garden or among the containers and boxes so they can encounter growing plants up close.
- Start with small plots, which are more manageable for younger children than large spaces. A small plot can be weeded and watered more easily by little hands, and small spaces also encourage ownership.
- Use signs. Even simple pictures will allow younger children to understand what is growing in the garden. Signs can also mark children's individual beds and plants so they can check on their progress throughout the season.

Using the Garden

PLANTING

❧ On planting day, it helps to have the seeds and seedlings laid out in advance close to where they will be planted, so children can focus on setting them into the prepared ground.

TENDING

❧ As the garden grows, make chores like watering more fun by cutting off the bottom of a large plastic bottle and "planting" the neck in the ground beside the plants. Children can fill the bottle with water from a watering can to add moisture to the soil.

HARVESTING & TASTING

❧ When it is time to harvest, some children love to eat as they pick, tasting pea pods, berries, or cherry tomatoes fresh from the vine. Consider planting a partial garden of finger foods to encourage tasting.

❧ After the harvest, try serving washed and thinly sliced raw foods with add-ons like a homemade light oil and vinegar dressing or yogurt-based ranch dressing for dipping.

❧ Use easy recipes to involve kids in preparing the vegetables—they'll often be willing to taste food they've helped prepare themselves.

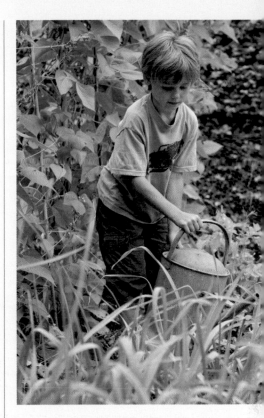

A LIVING CLASSROOM

Children's gardens teach lessons about the soil and the life cycle of plants and about where healthy food comes from. And they engage children of all ages with the green world around them.

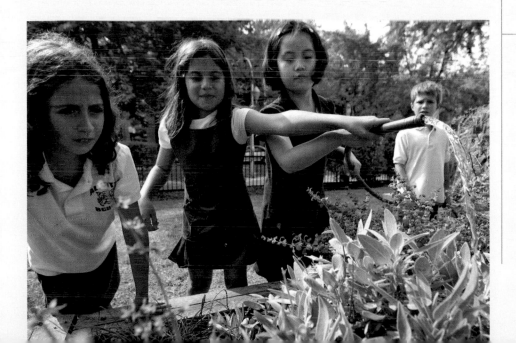

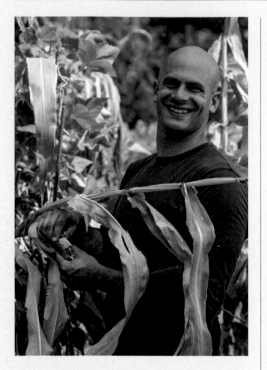

HARVESTING THE CORN
*Sam Kass and the other White House chefs take
great pleasure and pride in the food we grow
in our Kitchen Garden.*

Growing up, my family ate simple dinners together every night. I loved cooking with my parents, and while over time it became part of my weekly responsibilities, I never planned for cooking to become my life's passion or my vocation. But when I went to Vienna, Austria, during my last year in college, I got taken in by a chef who ended up teaching me most of what I know about food and cooking. For the next five years, I traveled, studied, and cooked. During that time, whether it was learning to make pasta with a grandmother in an Italian village or cooking five thousand tamales for the Day of the Dead celebration in Tlaxcala, Mexico, I experienced how food brings people together. I came to understand food not only as a crossroads of history, culture, and the daily enjoyment of eating, but also as a foundation of the environment, the economy, and our health.

My work in the White House Kitchen Garden has deepened my consciousness about the food we eat. Our garden has been connected to farmers from around the country, whose advice and wisdom have helped make the garden flourish. I have gotten a taste of their experience as I've worried about the peas shriveling or the lettuce failing to come up; what will we do if there is a late frost, an early snow, or too much rain? Through planting, harvesting, and working with farmers, I gained a greater appreciation and respect for the challenges of farming and risks that the men and women who grow this nation's food take when they sow a seed or harvest a crop. Growing food and coming to understand all that goes into bringing that food to our plates illuminates the real implications our food choices have for our health, our land, and our quality of life.

Just as the garden has broadened my horizons, the connection to growing food has changed the perspective of the kids who help the First Lady in the garden. The White House Kitchen Garden truly engages kids as active participants, giving them a chance to get their hands dirty and help create their own healthy, delicious meals. We have seen kids devour vegetables they previously turned up their noses at, or didn't even recognize, simply because they had a hand in planting or harvesting them. Raw rhubarb isn't exactly a tasty treat, but we've seen kids dance around chewing on it because they picked it themselves.

When kids help cook ingredients from the garden and transform them into delicious meals, they realize that ultimately, that's what gardening is about—it's about nourishing ourselves with delicious, healthy food. They come to understand that the food that is best for you has the best flavor. This experience can be truly transformative. It can affect their choices and habits for years to come. That is the essence of the White House Kitchen Garden and the First Lady's vision for this country.

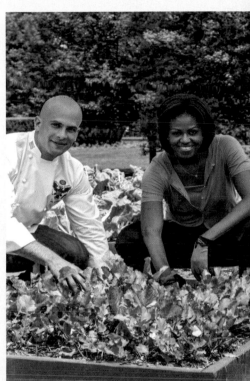

ENJOYING THE GARDEN
Above, "Each moment that we get to spend in the garden is a special privilege. It is a great opportunity to be part of something important, even life-changing."
—Chef Sam

TEACHABLE MOMENTS
Left, "We have had so many teachable moments in the garden, from planting through harvest. Nothing is more rewarding than watching children's faces light up with delight over a new plant or when they harvest something they have grown."
—Chef Sam

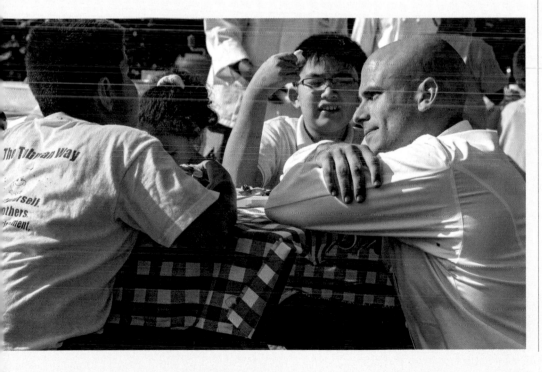

THE 2011

Fall Garden

PLAN

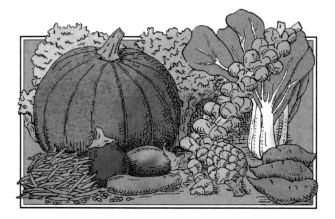

"When we engage children in harvesting our gardens—when we teach them about where their food comes from, how to prepare it, and how to grow it themselves—they reap the benefits well into the future."

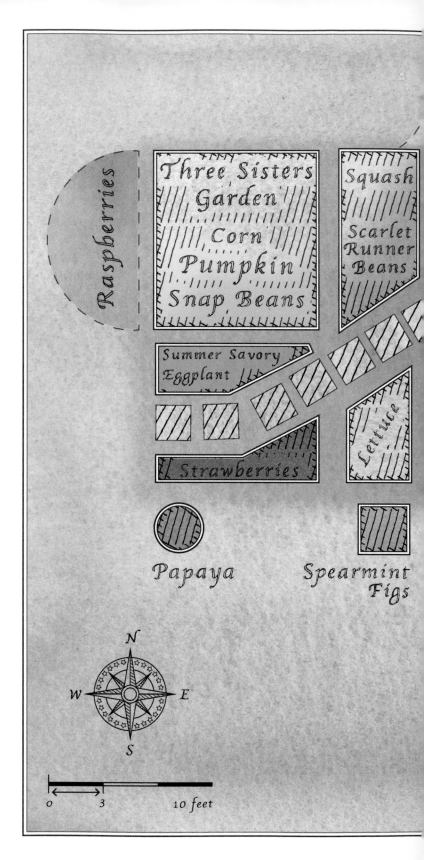

Raspberries

Three Sisters Garden
Corn
Pumpkin
Snap Beans

Squash
Scarlet Runner Beans

Summer Savory
Eggplant

Lettuce

Strawberries

Papaya

Spearmint
Figs

N
W   E
S

0   3   10 feet

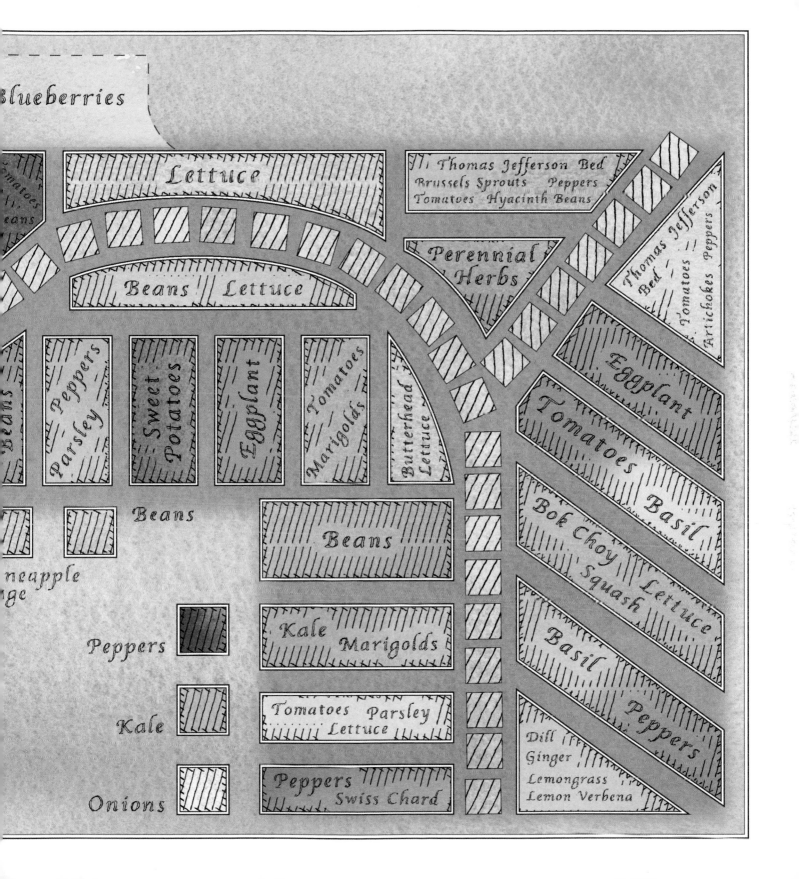

Blueberries

Lettuce

Thomas Jefferson Bed
Brussels Sprouts   Peppers
Tomatoes   Hyacinth Beans

Perennial
Herbs

Thomas Jefferson Bed

Tomatoes
Artichokes Peppers

Beans   Lettuce

Peppers
Parsley

Sweet
Potatoes

Eggplant

Tomatoes
Marigolds

Butterhead
Lettuce

Eggplant

Tomatoes
Basil

Beans

Bok Choy
Lettuce

Squash

Beans

Basil
Peppers

Kale   Marigolds

Peppers

Tomatoes   Parsley
Lettuce

Kale

Dill
Ginger
Lemongrass
Lemon Verbena

Onions

Peppers
Swiss Chard

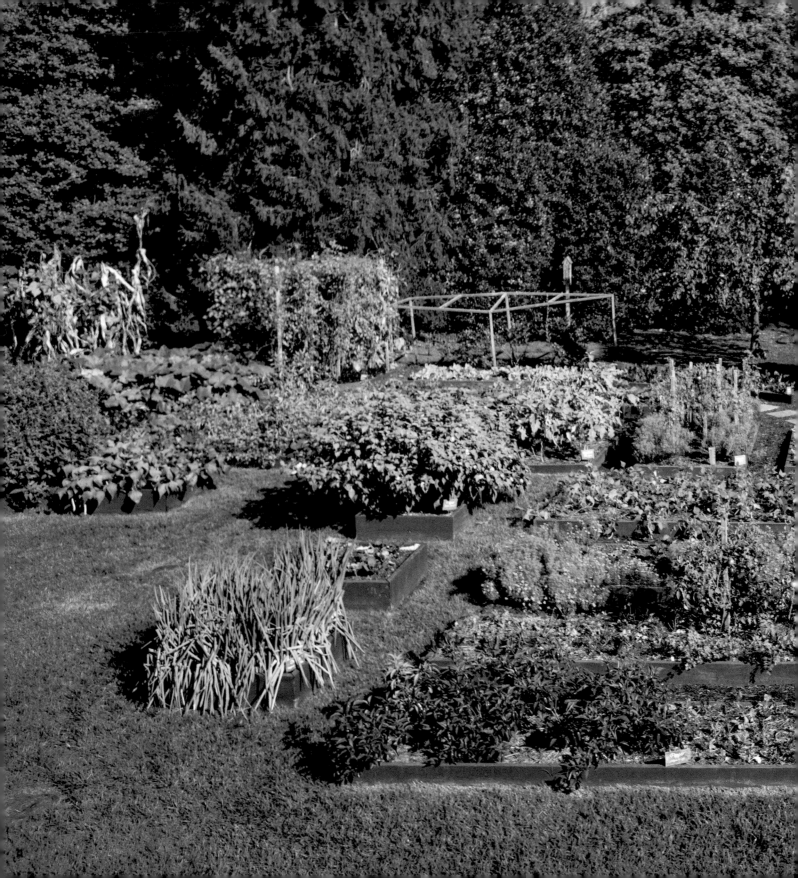

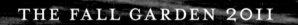
THE FALL GARDEN 2011

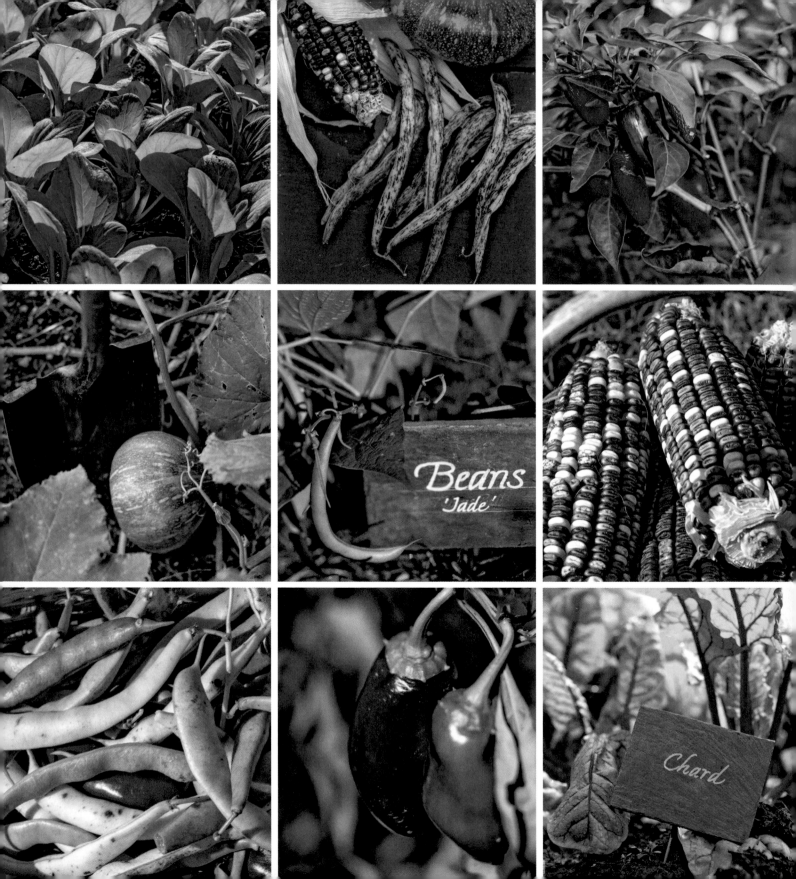

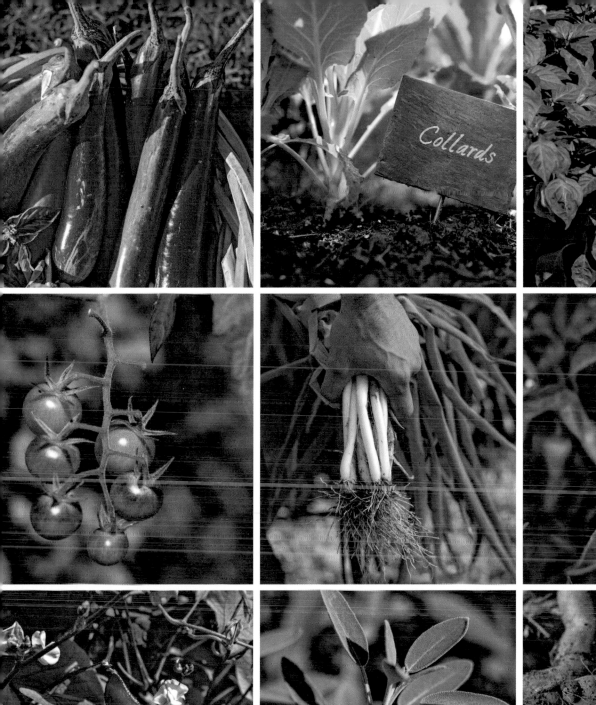
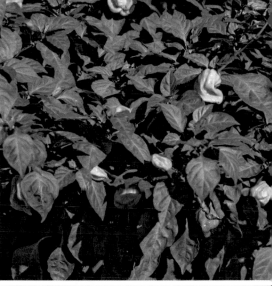
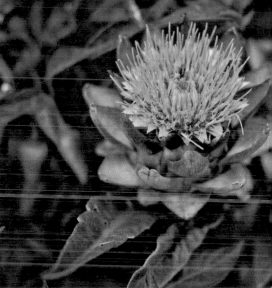
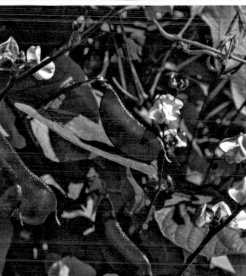
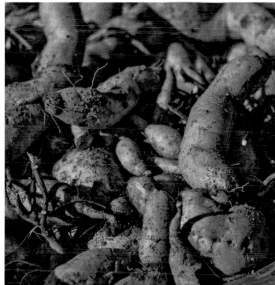

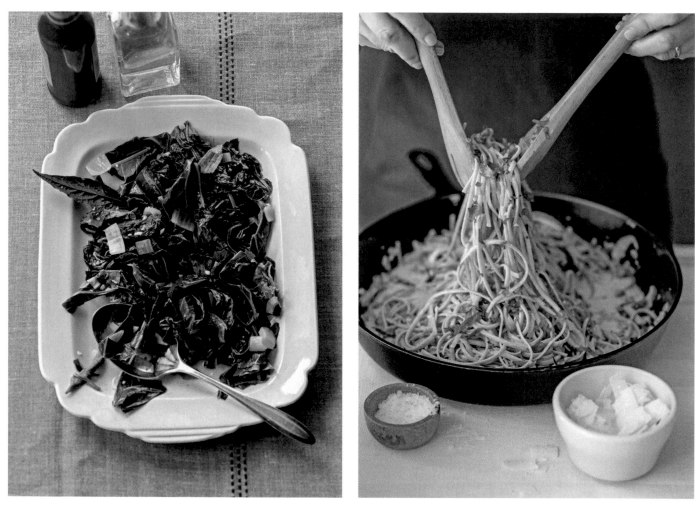

collard greens
page 241

linguine with
mushroom bacon sauce
page 242

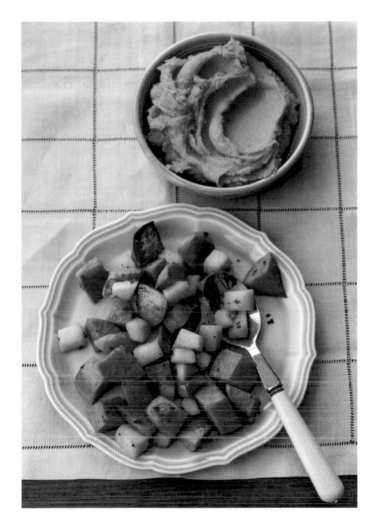

sweet potatoes two ways
page 244

sweet potato quick bread
page 246

FINAL THOUGHTS ON FALL

A good harvest is the result of months of effort, the culmination of what we've invested in our soil and our plants—and what we've invested in each other. As I have seen in the faces of the children who visit our garden and the guests at Miriam's Kitchen, the impact of just one harvest can extend far beyond our own tables. They and so many others have taught us that we most fully enjoy a good harvest by sharing it with others.

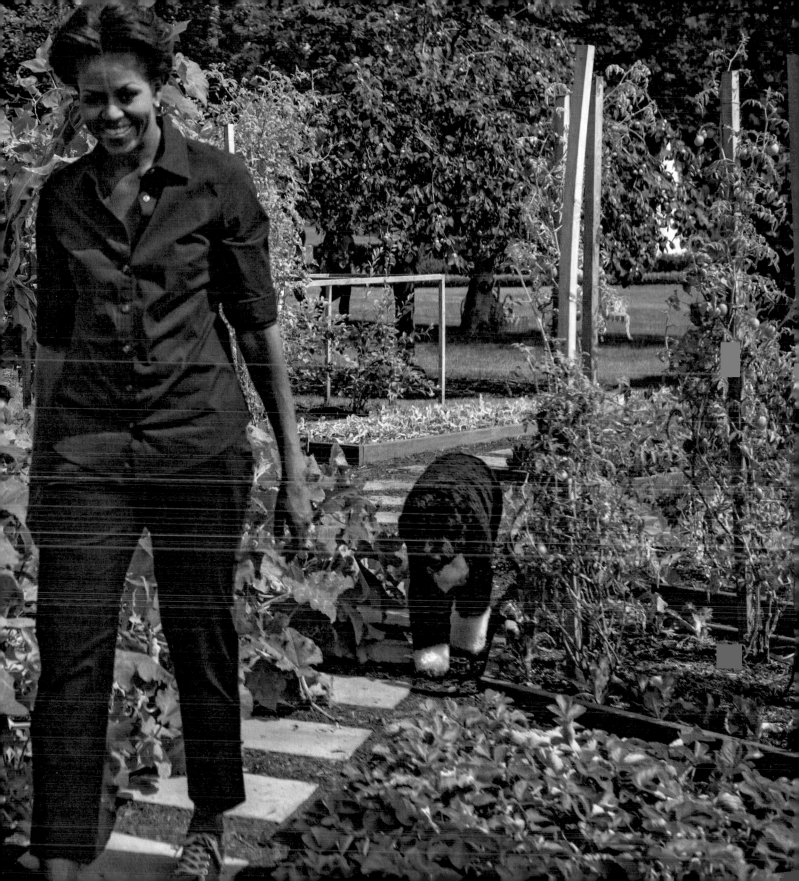

Winter

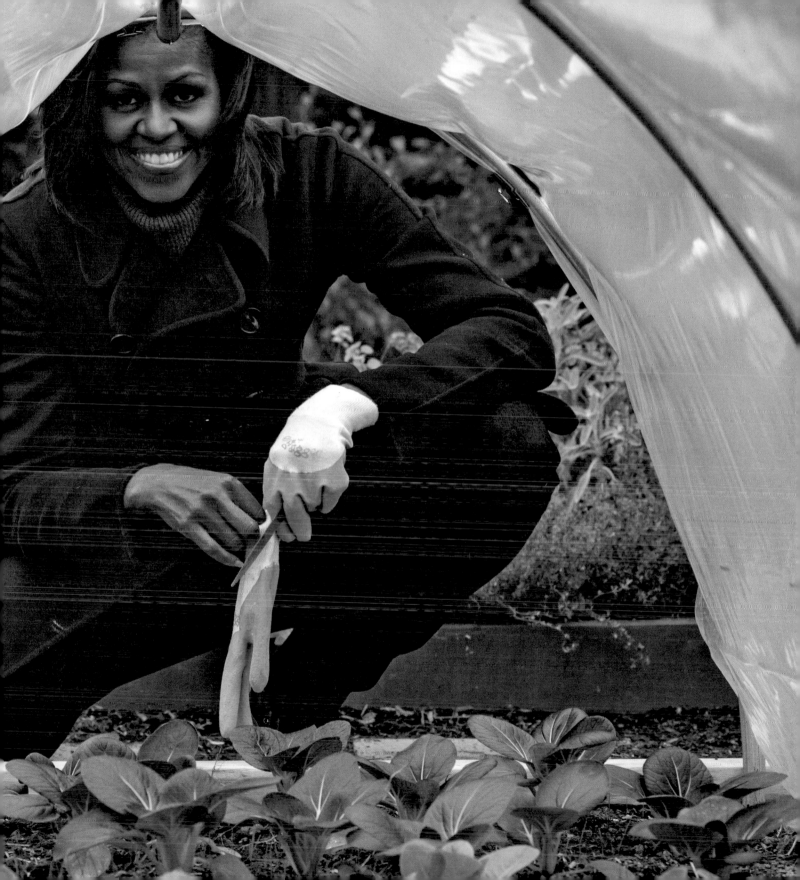

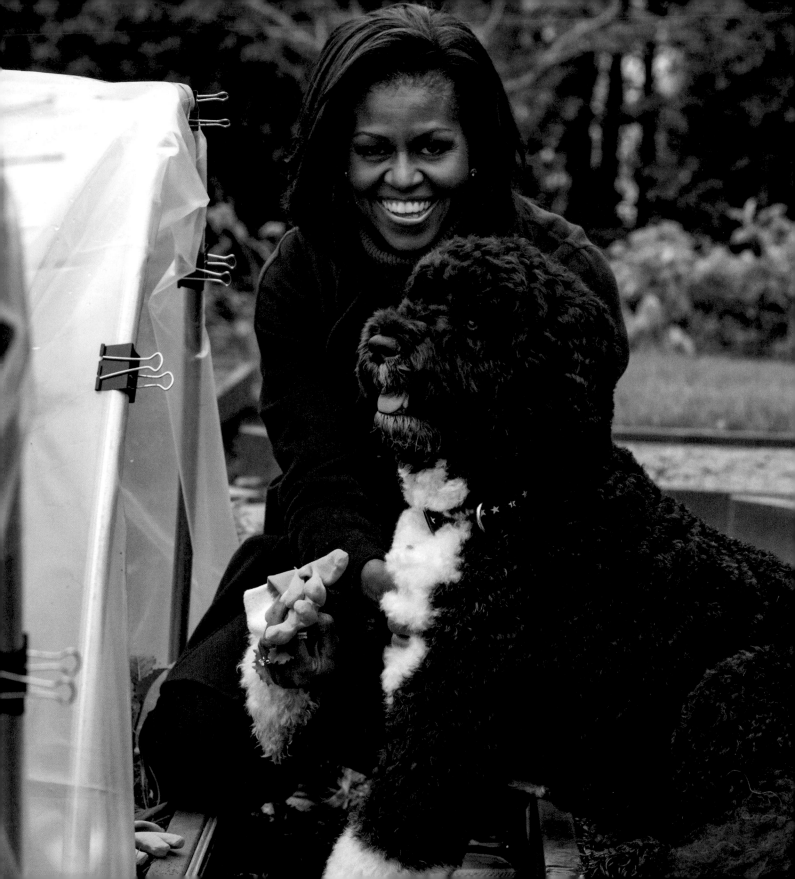

WINTER: GETTING CREATIVE AND BUILDING A FOUNDATION FOR SEASONS TO COME

Winter is a time for reflection, when we look back at the past year and marvel at how the tiny seeds we planted all those months ago blossomed into a thriving garden. Plummeting temperatures and drifting snow make gardening a challenge, but with ingenuity and hard work, we've been able to grow in ways we never thought possible. The same can be said of our work to build a healthier future for our children. Those first seeds we planted in our garden helped start a conversation that grew into a nationwide movement as people across this country united to address the challenge of childhood obesity. And together, with determination and creativity, we have begun building the foundation for a healthier generation and a healthier nation.

I originally assumed that after our fall harvest, we would have to wait until spring to resume growing our crops. I couldn't imagine how any of our vegetables would survive in temperatures that drop below freezing. I had heard that some farmers use a plastic covering to extend the growing season into the winter. But while I was intrigued by the prospect of keeping the garden alive, and I was open to experimenting, I was skeptical that a sheet of plastic would keep the plants warm through the D.C. winter.

In spite of my doubts, we went ahead and built what are called low tunnels, or hoop houses, simple metal frames that stand about two feet off the ground and are covered by a clear plastic tarp. To my amazement and delight, under those simple structures, several of our crops continued to flourish, even in very cold weather—and they were unusually sweet. I later learned that since sugars don't freeze, the plants produce a lot of sugars to protect themselves from the cold.

The lesson from that first winter was clear: In a garden, with a little ingenuity and imagination—and a whole lot of effort—you can achieve something you never thought possible.

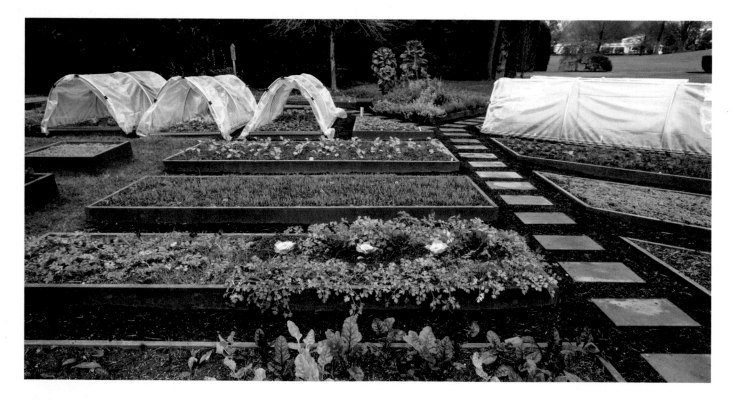

HOOP HOUSES:
A CREATIVE WINTER SOLUTION

As communities become dependent on local gardeners and farmers for more of their food, many are seeking to extend their growing season to provide more fresh produce and ensure that it is available all year round.

Hoop houses (also known as low tunnels) are a simple yet practical solution being employed by gardeners in places as cold as Maine. The plastic that covers the metal or wooden frame traps heat from the sun during the day. At night, when the temperature drops, the trapped heat keeps the plants from freezing. With the unpredictable weather in D.C., however, we have had some close calls. If we happen to have an unusually warm winter day, the tunnels can trap too much heat and turn into little ovens. To avoid baking our plants, we have to open the ends of the tunnels to let in the cool air and lower the temperature inside.

The Garden That Never Sleeps
Jim Adams, National Park Service Supervisory Horticulturist

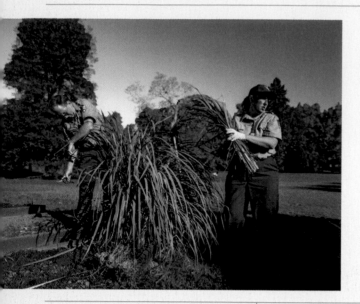

People tend to think of winter as a time when the growing world holds still, when the ground lies fallow, and there is little to do but wait for spring. But there is almost always activity in a garden, and if the soil has been well tended and well nourished, it is possible to grow and harvest plants even through the chill of the winter. We have been doing that for three years in the White House Kitchen Garden.

STARTING FRESH

"We never put the Kitchen Garden to bed; we are growing all year round. But at the start of winter, we clean out and nourish the beds. Planting for winter is like starting with a blank slate. Everything is new and anything is possible."
—Jim Adams

A year in the Kitchen Garden really starts in November; that's the time when we start fresh. As the lush, green South Lawn goes to sleep for the winter, we pull everything out from the garden beds except for the perennial herbs and the berry vines and bushes. All the remaining vegetable plants go in the compost bin. Then we add another layer of compost to the beds and cultivate the soil. We cover some of the beds with hoop houses, and in the rest we plant cover crops—plants like rye grass, winter wheat, or clover that prevent the soil from compacting in the winter from rain and snow. If you leave the soil bare, it almost always gets compacted, and it requires more work to prepare for the spring planting.

Winters have been a period of trial and error for our White House garden. The first year, we put up hoop houses where the garden had gotten the most sun in the summer, but we didn't realize how low the sun hangs in the sky during the winter season and how short its journey is from horizon to horizon. As a result, the big holly trees along the lower fence line blocked some of the late-day sun from our plants. But we still had a good harvest of lettuces and other greens that year, even with three major blizzards.

That snow taught us our second trial-and-error lesson. After the storms, we learned that we needed to set the hoop houses far enough apart so that we could shovel out any snow that accumulated. The next year, we repositioned the houses. That winter was less snowy but much colder. Ironically, we then struggled to keep the houses from getting too hot. It can get into the 80s inside the houses on a winter afternoon if it's a bright, sunny day, even if it was 30 or 32 degrees outside that morning. We'd often even have to open up the houses to let in the cold and lower the temperatures inside. Despite our challenges, many crops grew very well in the hoop houses. In fact, some varieties of lettuce grew even better in the hoop houses than during the regular garden season.

For me, one of the lessons of winter is that even when the trees are bare, when the lawn mowers have fallen silent, when the grass stays a perfect inch and a half high in a kind of frozen suspended animation, we never put the Kitchen Garden to bed. The garden thrives all year round.

Winter is also when we begin to plan for the future, preparing our seedlings for the spring planting and eagerly anticipating the next season, the next planting, and the next harvest.

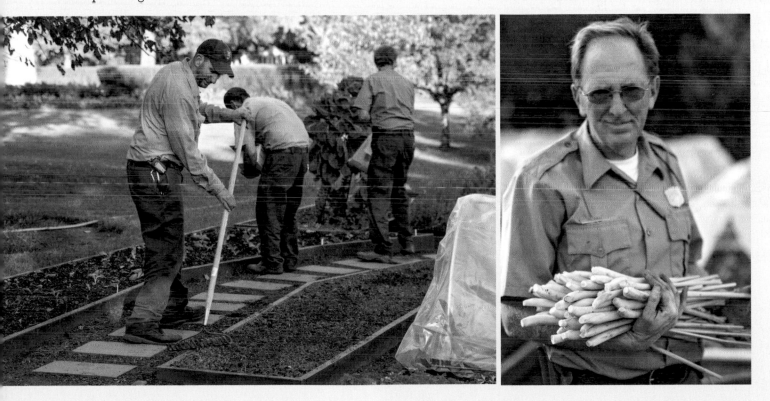

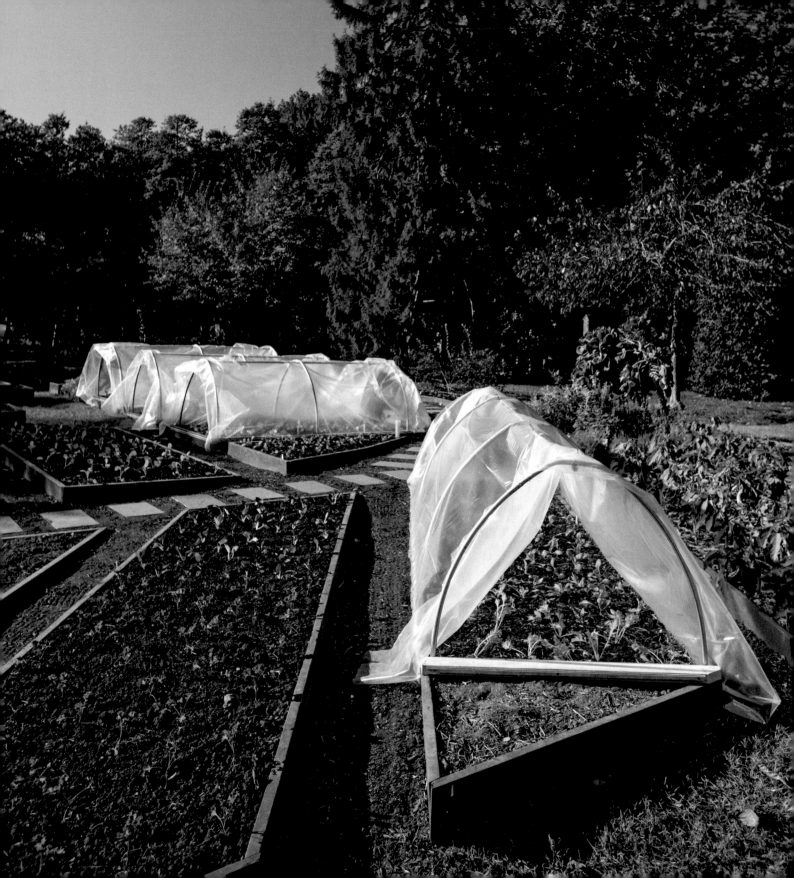

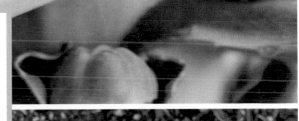

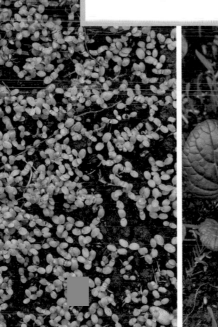

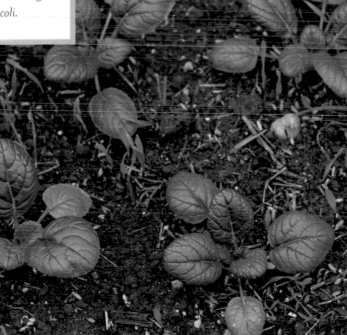

COLD-WEATHER
SURVIVORS

*It's entirely possible to harvest your
garden throughout the winter, if you start
with the right plants. The following are
safe bets for cold weather: spinach, kale,
chard, mustard greens, collards,
bok choy (a tender Chinese cabbage),
lettuce, and broccoli.*

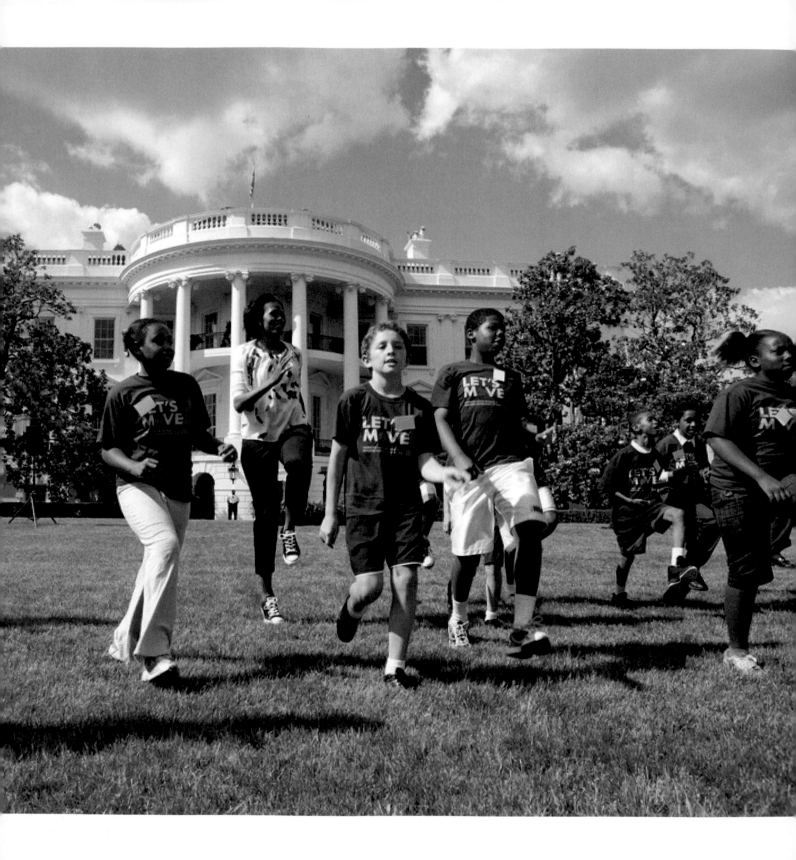

The Challenge of Childhood Obesity

Much like growing a garden in the winter, at first the challenge of child-hood obesity seemed insurmountable. Over the past three decades, child-hood obesity rates in America have tripled, and today nearly one in three children are overweight or obese. And these numbers don't even paint the full picture. This isn't about inches and pounds and how our kids look. It's about how they feel and how they feel about themselves; and it's about the impact we're seeing on every aspect of their lives.

Pediatricians are seeing more and more kids with diseases like high blood pressure and type 2 diabetes that we used to see only in adults, and today one in three children are on track to develop diabetes at some point in their lives. Teachers are seeing teasing and bullying; school counselors are seeing depression and low self-esteem; and coaches are seeing kids struggling to keep up or stuck on the sidelines. Studies have even shown that what our kids eat and how active they are can affect their performance on standardized tests.

All of this doesn't just affect our children's success—it affects the success of our country as well. It affects our economy. We currently spend nearly $150 billion a year to treat obesity-related health conditions, and obesity can impact everything from worker productivity to employee absenteeism. Believe it or not, obesity can also even affect our national security. Military leaders report that obesity is now one of the most common disqualifiers for military service, and today more than one-quarter of our nation's seventeen- to twenty-four-year-olds are actually too overweight to serve in our military.

In January 2010, I had the privilege of visiting South Carolina's Fort Jackson, the largest Army basic training center in the nation, where I met Lieutenant General Mark Hertling, who gave me a briefing on just how dire the situation is.

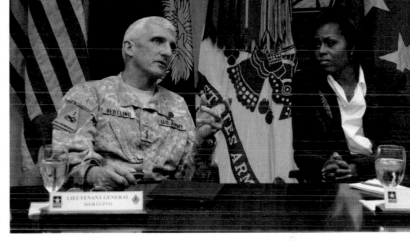

VISITING FORT JACKSON
During my visit to Fort Jackson, Lieutenant General Mark Hertling told me about how our military is leading the way to encourage healthy eating and healthier lifestyles.

A CHALLENGE FOR ALL OF US
Lieutenant General Mark Hertling

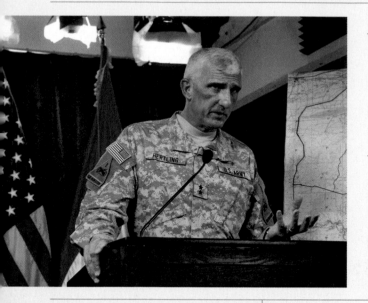

Around 2006, we began to see a sharp decrease in physical capability among the young civilians applying to join the Army, and then we saw that these recruits were more likely to sustain bone and deep-muscle injuries during basic training. We soon made the connection that many of these soldiers had attended elementary and high school in the mid- and late 1990s, when physical education had been eliminated from the curriculum in many states.

Of the Army's 129,000 applicants every year, a staggering 41 percent are overweight or obese. After years of consuming too many carbonated drinks and sugary snacks and consuming too little milk and calcium, most of our soldiers have brittle bones, and 62 percent of our new soldiers need significant dental repair to their teeth before they can deploy. And while in 2004, only 4 percent of male recruits and 10.5 percent of female recruits failed the Army's Entry Physical Fitness Test (which requires one minute of push-ups, one minute of sit-ups, and a one-mile run), by 2010 those numbers had exploded: 46.7 percent of males and 54.6 percent of females were failing that exact same test. That means that in half a decade, in just five years, we have moved from a nation in which fewer than 10 percent of recruits cannot pass a basic fitness test to a nation in which roughly 50 percent of recruits cannot pass that same test.

As a result of poor diet and a lack of exercise in schools and homes, when they begin to exercise, new recruits often have serious bone-density issues, making them prone to stress fractures and other injuries. In 2008, at Fort Jackson alone, we had 135 cases of major femoral bone and hip injuries.

These injuries cost $100,000 to $300,000 each to repair and in some cases, they even end a soldier's career. Today, the Army is spending millions of dollars to treat injuries like these, and we're hiring more dentists to repair our recruits' teeth.

While we can get our soldiers in shape during basic training and keep them in shape while they serve, another problem remains: How do we also improve health in the soldier's family—their spouse and children—and then how do we ensure a healthy lifestyle is passed to the next generation? How do we change our behavior and our culture before it contributes to early onset of diabetes, coronary disease, osteoporosis, and even psychological difficulties? How do we do all this before it is truly too late?

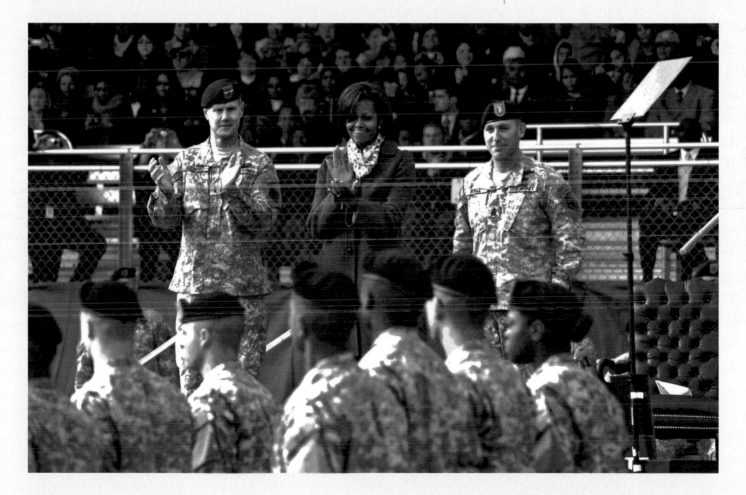

How We Got Here

We didn't arrive here overnight. It took decades for us to reach this moment when so many of our children face such a serious threat to their health and well-being. And in order to solve this problem, it's important to understand how we got here in the first place.

Back when many of us were growing up, our society was structured so that healthy eating and exercise were natural parts of our lives. We didn't even have to think about it—that was just the way it was. There were only a few channels on TV, and kids' cartoons were mostly on Saturday mornings, not broadcast at all hours, every day of the week. When *American Bandstand* and

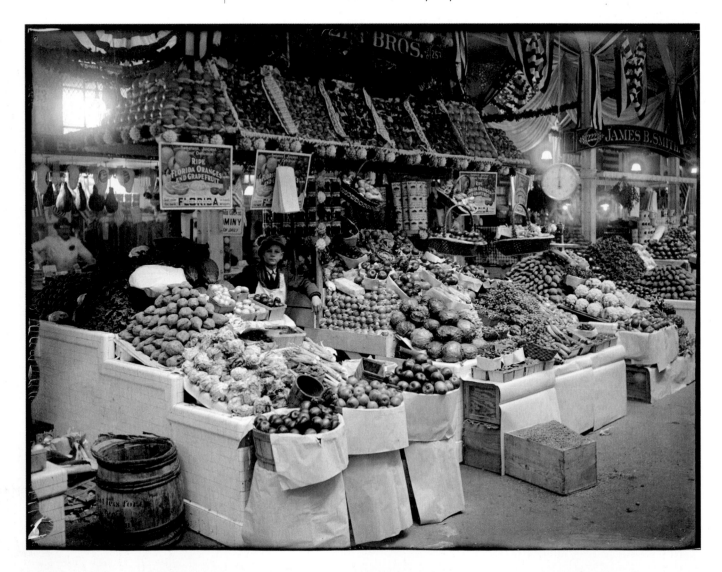

Soul Train ended, we headed out to play. We didn't come home until it was time for dinner—and we usually ate that dinner around the kitchen table, as a family. My family hardly ever ate out—and I can remember only a handful of times when we got takeout. My brother and I got to have pizza a few times a year, mostly as a reward for good grades on our report cards. And I'll never forget the time we were allowed to have take-out food at my grandmother's house. We spent many weekends with her, and we often begged her to let us have burgers and fries from around the corner. Finally, one lunchtime, she relented. My brother and I looked at each other wide-eyed. We couldn't believe she had given in.

One of my uncles went out to pick up the cheeseburgers and fries, and when he returned, my grandmother intercepted him, snatched the bags out of his hands, and took them straight into the kitchen. She unwrapped the burgers and put them on our plates. Then she carefully laid out the fries beside them. And then, much to our horror, she opened up a can of peas and promptly served us two scoops each. Take-out food or not, my grandma believed in feeding her family a balanced meal at *every* meal, and she couldn't feed her grandchildren a proper lunch if it didn't have at least one vegetable.

Kids today lead very different lives. They can watch pretty much whatever they want whenever they want on TV. While a generation ago, three-quarters of our kids went outside every day to play, now only about one quarter of them do. And only about 15 percent—fewer than one in five—of our high schoolers get the recommended one hour of physical activity a day.

Our eating habits have also changed. Today, fresh food is often more expensive than convenience food. Parents are also working harder and harder to make ends meet, and they often just don't have the time or the energy to make the kind of home-cooked meals we grew up with. When they do cook, many find that with all the brands and products out there, it's hard to know which foods are healthy and which ones aren't. And many families don't have a single store selling fresh food in their community, so even if they want to purchase healthy foods, they can't. Taken together, the impact of these factors on our kids' health—and on their prospects in life—is sobering.

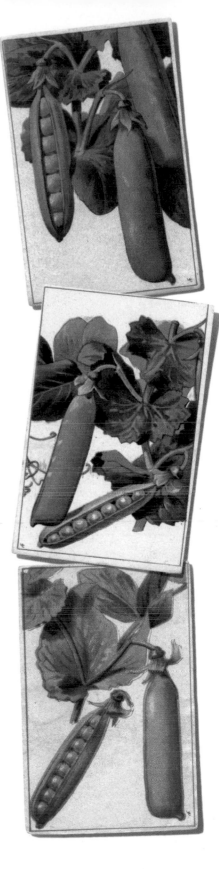

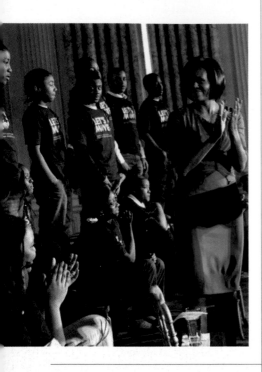

Launching *Let's Move!*

It was clear from the beginning that restoring our children's health would be no small challenge. Just as we didn't arrive at this moment overnight, we can't expect to find some quick fix or magic pill that will change us back overnight. I knew the conventional wisdom on this issue, particularly when it comes to changing how our kids eat. There's the assumption that kids don't like healthy food, so why try to feed it to them? There's the belief that healthy food doesn't sell as well, so companies will never change the products they offer. And there's the sense that this problem is so big, and so entrenched, that no matter what we do, we'll never be able to solve it.

But here's what gave me hope: the simple fact that we all love our children, and none of us wants this kind of future for them or for our country. None of us wants our kids to live diminished lives because we failed to step up today. We don't want them looking back decades from now and asking us, "Why didn't you help us when you had a chance? Why didn't you put us first when it mattered most?"

And the more I learned about this problem, the more I came to believe that we could solve it. This isn't like putting a man on the moon or inventing the cell phone. It doesn't take some stroke of genius or feat of technology. We have everything we need, right now, to help our kids lead healthy lives. Rarely in the history of this country have we encountered a problem of such magnitude and consequence that is so eminently solvable. So instead of just talking about this issue, or worrying and wringing our hands about it, we decided to get moving.

On February 9, 2010, in the middle of two huge Washington, D.C., snowstorms, we launched *Let's Move!* While our goal was ambitious, the idea behind *Let's Move!* was very simple: that all of us—parents and teachers; doctors and coaches; business, faith, and community leaders; and others—have a role to play in helping our kids lead healthier lives. We know government doesn't have all the answers; and there is no one-size-fits-all program or policy that will solve this problem. Every family and every community is different, and each of us needs to find solutions that fit with our own budgets, needs, and tastes.

We also know that we need to attack this problem from every angle,

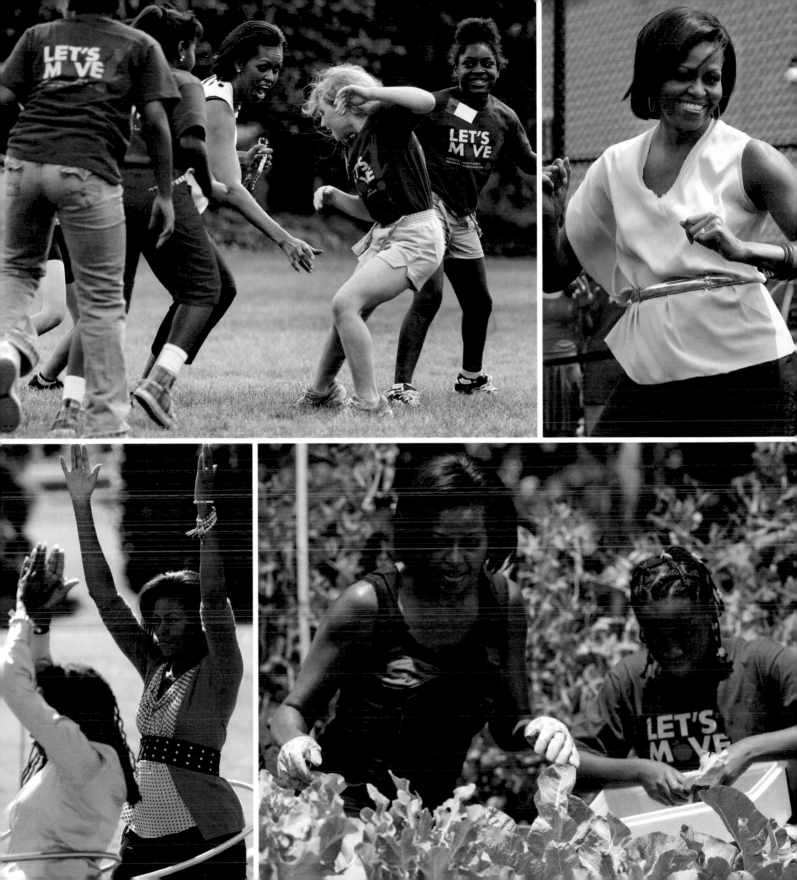

because we can serve kids the healthiest school lunches imaginable, but if there's no supermarket in their community, and they don't have nutritious food at home, then they still won't have a healthy diet. We can build shiny new supermarkets on every block, but if parents don't have the information they need, they'll still struggle to make healthy choices for their kids. And if kids aren't active, then no matter how well we feed them, they still won't be leading healthy lives.

We decided to focus our efforts on five key areas:

1. Creating a healthy start for children in their earliest years
2. Empowering parents and caregivers with information to make healthy choices for their children
3. Helping our schools support our children's health
4. Ensuring that all families have access to healthy, affordable food
5. Finding new ways for our kids to get moving and rediscover active play

Giving Our Children a Healthy Start

In the past few decades, obesity rates among kids ages two to five have doubled. And a recent study of nearly two hundred overweight or obese children found that more than half of them first became overweight before their second birthday. Today some children as young as three already show early warning signs for heart disease.

Because we know how formative those early years can be, we launched *Let's Move! Child Care.* Ranging from small home-based facilities to national organizations like Head Start and Bright Horizons, child-care providers care for more than half of all kids under the age of five. And many of them are

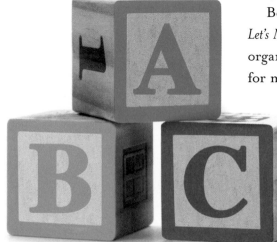

now rethinking the meals and snacks they serve and the activities they offer. They're replacing sugary drinks with water, low-fat milk, and 100 percent fruit juice. They're replacing hours in front of the TV with hours spent running around outside. And they're teaching kids to make healthy choices for themselves, instilling good habits that can last a lifetime.

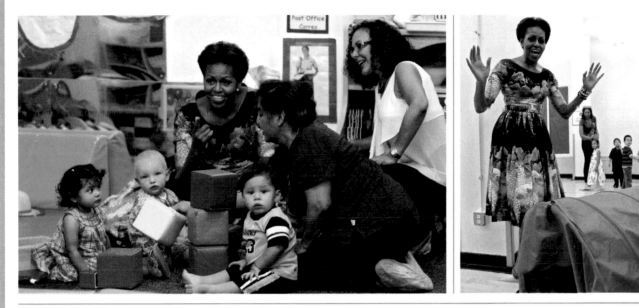

In June 2011, I had the pleasure of visiting CentroNía, a child-care facility in Washington, D.C., that has taken all kinds of steps to give their kids a healthy start. They cook their meals on-site, using local fruits and vegetables as often as possible, and they serve food family-style and teach the kids what healthy portion sizes look like. They've planted a garden and built a playground on their roof, and they take the kids to play in local parks and community spaces as often as possible.

As a result of these changes, CentroNía's nurse has seen far fewer kids visiting her office with stomachaches. The staff has also noticed that more children are willing to try new foods. And since the kids like what they try, they've been asking their parents to serve healthy foods at home as well.

LET'S MOVE! CHILD CARE CHECKLIST

- One to two hours of physical activity a day

- Limit screen time for all kids and eliminate it for kids under two

- Serve a fruit or vegetable at every meal

- Serve only water, low-fat milk, or 100 percent juice

- Support mothers who choose to breastfeed

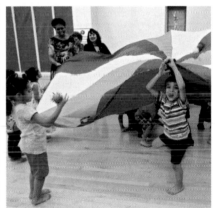

A CENTRONÍA DAY
Active play and healthy food are very important for young children. At CentroNía, kids get plenty of both.

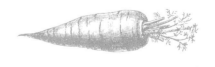

Empowering Parents to Make Healthy Choices

As parents, we want to do everything we can to keep our kids healthy. But kids don't come with an instruction manual. And as parents we're bombarded with contradictory information at every turn, and we don't always know who or what to believe.

I know what that's like, because I've been there. I haven't always lived in the White House. It wasn't that long ago that I was a working mom, dashing from meetings and conference calls to ballet recitals and the car-pool pickup line. And when it came time to do the grocery shopping each week, I would walk up and down those aisles searching high and low for the best options for my family, struggling to figure out which foods were healthy and which ones weren't.

I know that many other parents have had a similar experience. We want to buy healthy food, but it can sometimes be hard to find—and afford— products that are good for our kids and taste good too.

That's why through *Let's Move!*, we're working with businesses and organizations across America to give parents the information and opportunities they need to make healthier choices for their families. In June 2011, the United States Department of Agriculture partnered with more than fifty-seven hundred organizations—from churches and hospitals to grocery stores and schools—to launch and promote our new MyPlate/ MiPlato initiative. MyPlate, which has replaced the old food pyramid, is an easy-to-understand icon that makes eating well simple. It's divided into five sections: Fruits, Vegetables, Grains, Protein, and Dairy. And as long as you're eating reasonable portion sizes in the recommended proportions, then you're in good shape.

We're also working with major American companies, restaurants, and retailers, supporting their efforts to produce and sell healthier, more affordable food. Over the past two years, national food manufacturers have committed to cutting 1.5 trillion calories from their products. Darden Restaurants, the world's largest full-service restaurant com-

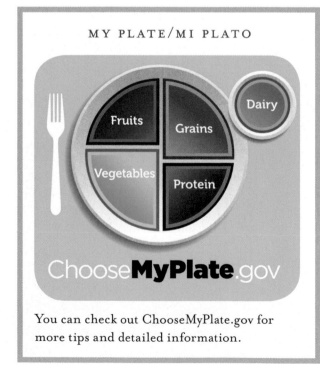

MY PLATE/MI PLATO

You can check out ChooseMyPlate.gov for more tips and detailed information.

pany, whose brands include Red Lobster and Olive Garden, is reducing calories and salt and revamping their kids' menus to offer healthier choices. Walmart is providing a special seal to help parents identify healthy food products, making options like fresh produce more affordable, and working to cut sugar and salt and eliminate trans-fats from the products they sell.

ONE FAMILY'S SUCCESS WITH MYPLATE

In February 2012, I had the pleasure of having dinner with Kern and Patrice Halls and their two young sons, Keian and Kamryn, at their home in Ocoee, Florida. Kern used MyPlate to transform his diet—and his family's—and they were all eating better and feeling healthier as a result.

"A few months ago, I went to my doctor for my annual checkup, and he was very blunt with me about how I had the recipe for disaster: I ate poorly, was overweight, didn't work out, and had a lot of stress in my life. So he asked me if I wanted to be on medicine the rest of my life, die early, or commit to making some adjustments. Needless to say, I chose the latter, and I started changing the way I—and my family—ate.

"I went through my cabinets and freezers and donated items that did not match up with the food groups in the new MyPlate. We also started to exercise together as a family, taking family walks and bike rides. And on Sundays, we now prepare for the week by cutting and bagging up fresh fruits in ready-to-eat portions—we consume many more fruits and veggies this way.

"The new MyPlate was so simple to use and follow that it made these changes easy. So far, I have lost fifteen pounds—and my wife has lost weight as well—and I am on my way back to my military weight (and I left the Navy more than a decade ago!). Most important, we've learned to 'eat to live' rather than 'live to eat,' and I now feel that I can pass healthy habits on to my boys and on to generations to come. If it was not for MyPlate, the chances of my very existence on earth today would be slim to none."

—KERN HALLS

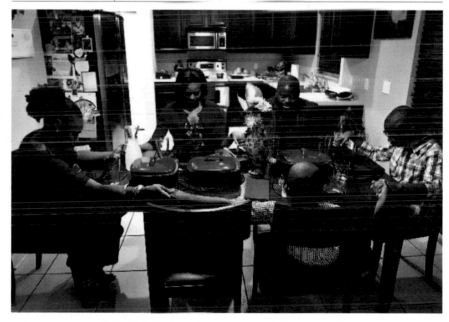

The Halls family and me saying grace before our meal.

Building Healthy Schools for All Our Children

In 1966, when President Johnson signed legislation expanding the National School Lunch Program to include school breakfasts and meals at preschools, he declared, "Good nutrition is essential to good learning."

That sentiment is equally true today. We know that the food our kids eat can affect their academic performance, and one study found that obese children are actually more likely to miss more than two weeks of school a year. So when more than thirty-one million American children are getting up to half their calories each day from school breakfasts and lunches, it is critical—not just for their health, but for their success in school—that we make those meals as nutritious as possible.

So I was thrilled when, in December 2010, my husband signed into law the Healthy, Hunger-Free Kids Act. This act sets higher standards for food served in schools, and for the first time it sets standards for food sold in vending machines and à la carte lines as well. In addition, for the first time in thirty years, schools will get more of the resources and support they need to meet these standards.

Because of this act, schools will soon be providing more fruits, vegeta-

THE HEALTHY, HUNGER-FREE KIDS ACT

Standing beside my husband for the signing of this historic legislation. It was a proud day for me and a significant step forward for the health of our nation's children.

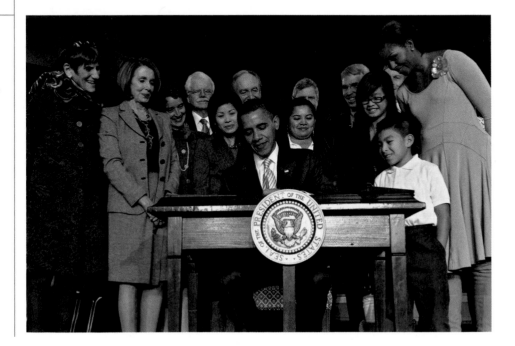

bles, and whole grains, along with low-fat milk (and any flavored milk must be fat free). The act also ensures that more children who are eligible for free and reduced-price meals are actually receiving those meals, because for kids whose families are struggling, school meals are often their main—or only—source of nutrition.

But even before we passed this new law, schools across the country were already rethinking the food they served and finding new ways for students to be active during the day. Between 2009 and 2012, participation in the HealthierUS School Challenge—a USDA program recognizing schools that serve healthy food and provide opportunities for physical activity—jumped from 625 schools to nearly 3,000. These schools—and so many others—have gotten creative. They're holding taste tests and recipe contests. They're partnering with local farmers to get fresh food into their lunchrooms and teach kids about where their food comes from. And through our *Chefs Move! to Schools* program, more than thirty-four hundred chefs—including our White House chefs—have signed up to volunteer in local schools. Every day, these chefs are planting school gardens, teaching kids about healthy eating, and helping cafeteria staffs transform their menus with recipes that are nutritious and taste good too.

A BETTER SCHOOL LUNCH
In January 2012, at Alexandria, Virginia's Parklawn Elementary School, I helped unveil new USDA guidelines for school lunches. Now parents can be confident that when their kids go to school, they will be getting the nutritious food they need to learn and grow.

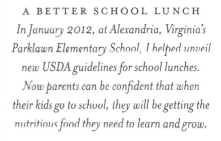

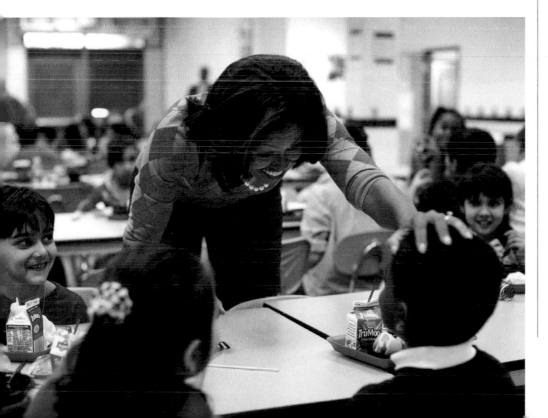

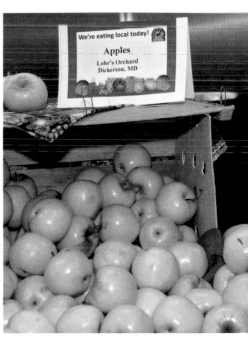

THE FARM GOES TO SCHOOL

BOSTON, MASSACHUSETTS

What began in 2008 as a pilot project to get Massachusetts-grown food into six school cafeterias in Boston is now in all forty-six full-service kitchens in the Boston public schools. Every Thursday is Local Lunch Thursday, featuring vegetables and fruits grown by farmers in western Massachusetts. Kids are offered vegetable medleys of carrots, butternut squash, and rutabaga, as well as green beans, collard greens, apples, fresh strawberries, and coleslaw made with locally grown cabbages.

Over time, the program has found creative ways to meet the challenges of school cooking. Every day, cafeteria staffs have to prepare and serve hundreds of meals quickly, with some students having only twenty minutes total to stand in line and eat their lunch. To help Local Lunch Thursdays succeed, the school district's farmer partner does much of the vegetable prep at the farm and ships a precut vegetable medley ready for roasting in the school ovens.

Kim Szeto, the Farm to School coordinator for Boston, encourages students to try these locally grown vegetables by handing out samples in the cafeterias. She explains, "We often bring the whole vegetable or seedling into the cafeteria along with the samples to show students. The more kids know about these vegetables, the more they might like to eat them and even to grow them."

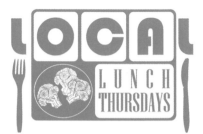

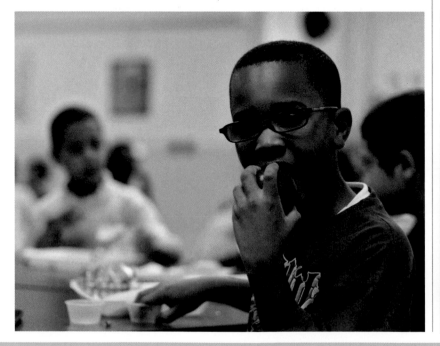

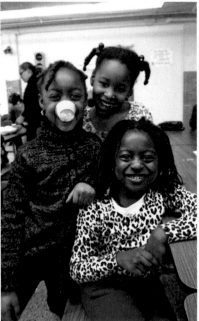

SHAWNEE, OKLAHOMA

At three elementary schools in Shawnee, Oklahoma, family farmers Claudia and Ricky Crow arrive in the fall with a trailer filled with pie pumpkins, one for each child. Claudia explains how the pumpkins grow from small seeds, and the kids have a chance to roast these seeds and take home recipes for things like pumpkin meatloaf. Of her experience working in schools, Claudia says:

"I wanted to get involved with the schools when I started noticing that fewer and fewer families with young children were coming to shop in the farmers' markets. When I talk to kids, they are shocked that they couldn't have a hamburger or eat a pizza without a farmer. I've met kids who can't guess what a red potato is when they see it because the only time they've seen potatoes is as French fries, Tater Tots, or in some kind of instant mash.

"When I ask kids how many of them want to be farmers, no hands go up—they don't seem to consider farming a viable profession. I hope we can change that. I always take a bag of soil with me when I visit a school. I explain that while dirt is something you want to brush off, soil is something you want to preserve for generations. You want to care for it and nurture it. And hopefully we can grow some more farmers with it too."

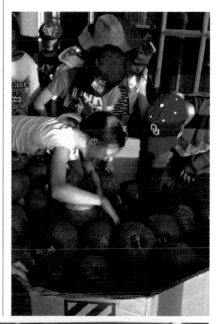

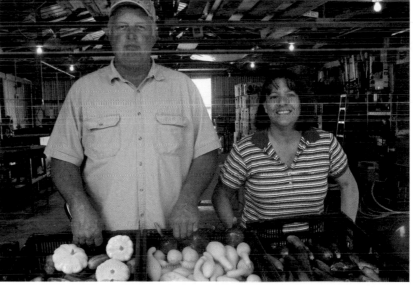

CLAUDIA AND RICKY CROW
Claudia and Ricky Crow began donating their time at schools when they realized how few children had ever met a farmer. "For many of the kids, any time spent with a farmer is an eye-opening experience," explains Deborah Taylor, coordinator of Shawnee, Oklahoma's nutrition and food services. "Some kids are shocked to see dirt on a vegetable; they say 'Ew, yuck,' because they didn't know the food was grown in soil."

Teachable Moments at School Salad Bars

In November 2010, I visited Riverside Elementary School in the Little Havana section of Miami, Florida. Riverside was the first school in the nation to get a salad bar through *Salad Bars 2 Schools*, a special initiative that *Let's Move!* supported to put six thousand salad bars in schools. We brought a group of fifth-grade kids into the cafeteria, where we had laid out bowls of vegetables, each of which would be part of the salad bar. The kids then went from table to table touching and tasting the vegetables. As I walked around, I realized that many of these kids had never even seen some of these vegetables before. They held them, looked them over, and were almost afraid to taste them at first. One little boy ran up to me to show me different ingredients he was considering including in his salad and asked, "Can I eat this? Can I eat that?" Today, thanks to the efforts of schools across the country, millions of children are learning the answer to those questions.

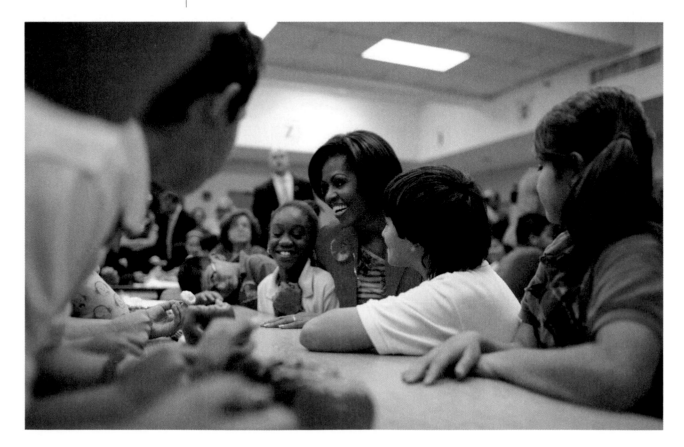

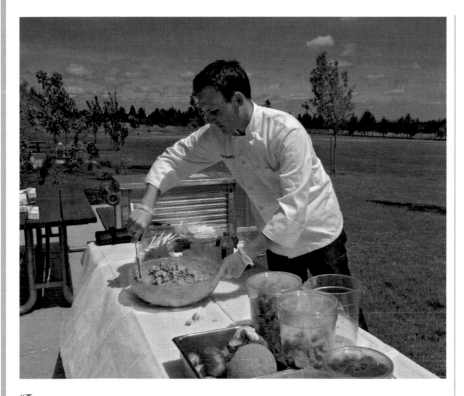

with Greek yogurt and honey, and an opportunity to taste different herbs.

"Students often have little exposure to raw ingredients. They don't know what a sweet potato looks like. They haven't seen food in all its stages, from raw, to prep, to final—and sometimes they're reluctant to taste something new. But I love that moment when they finally agree to try something they were suspicious of, and take that first bite really reluctantly, and then suddenly realize that they actually like it. I love seeing their faces light up and hearing them say, 'Yum.' That is a truly amazing experience."

—CHEF GARRETT BERDAN

"I got involved with *Chefs Move! to Schools* because I wanted to do a volunteer project in my community. One of the local elementary schools was participating in a Department of Agriculture grant program that offers kids an afternoon snack of fruit and vegetables. I decided to try making baked kale chips for the kids as part of that program. I started off by showing the kids the whole leaf of raw, green kale, which is big and prehistoric looking, and I swished the leaves around so that they could hear the sounds they made. Then I brought out a big tub of baked kale chips and shook it, which sounds like dry autumn leaves crunching. That way, the kids could hear the difference between raw and cooked kale. I then invited the kids to taste the kale chips, and almost all of them did. Most loved them. I got high fives and fist bumps. Kids came back for seconds. Suddenly, kale didn't seem like a big, scary green vegetable anymore. And we've had other successful projects since then, including a fruit salad

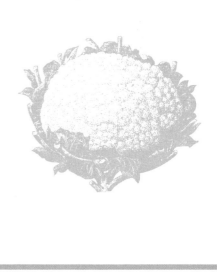

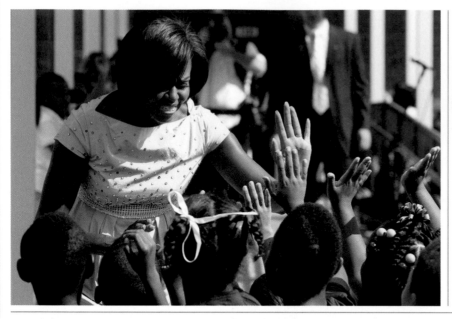

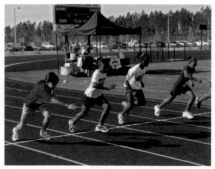

ST. TAMMANY PARISH,
SLIDELL, LOUISIANA
In 2010, I had a chance to see the kids in Slidell "Go, Glow, and Grow." Their schools are working to be among the healthiest in the nation.

In September 2010, I visited Slidell, Louisiana, which is in St. Tammany parish. Slidell was one of the areas hardest hit by Hurricane Katrina, but five years later, they had not only rebuilt their schools and neighborhoods, they had begun to transform the health of their children and families as well. As school superintendent Trey Folse explains, "It started with the food service program, and the kids and teachers jumped on board, and then the parents."

Schools started serving fruit for dessert—"Cookies are definitely not the norm around here anymore," adds Folse. They also began looking for ways to add more whole grains—white rice was replaced with brown rice, for example—and more fruits and vegetables as well. "We came up with healthier gumbo recipes, and our goal is soon to cook most of the school meals from scratch," says Folse. In addition, they created a nutritional program called Go, Glow, and Grow. "Go" is for the whole-grain foods that provide healthy carbohydrates; "glow" is for the vegetables and fruits that are high in vitamins and minerals; and "grow" is for the protein-rich foods that help build muscles.

To complement their new eating plan, the school district began focusing on fitness as well. They hosted an elementary school track meet, and a local football stadium was packed with parents watching their children compete. The best athletes went on to a statewide meet at Louisiana State University, where on their first try the team from Slidell came in fourth. Now Slidell kids "want to jump and sprint rather than sit in front of video games," says Folse, and teachers report that kids who exercise are better prepared to learn the next day at school.

In 2005, Cypress Cove Elementary School in Slidell was the first school in the nation to receive the highest award in the HealthierUS School Challenge. By 2010, all of the St. Tammany elementary schools had received the highest award in the challenge—the Gold Award of Distinction.

BUILD A BETTER LUNCH
Advice from Executive Chef (and Mom) Cris Comerford

As the mother of a ten-year-old, I'm always trying to think up new ways to make sure my daughter is getting a healthy and appealing lunch. And as a chef, I have to work extra hard to make sure that I'm eating balanced meals at lunch too rather than just snacking on whatever food I'm preparing that day. But I've learned that all of us—adults and kids—can build a better lunch with just a few small steps:

Choose fruits, veggies, and lean proteins. Fresh fruit, like an apple, an orange, or grapes, is always a good choice; if fruit is canned or in syrup, check to make sure there is no added sugar. Sliced turkey or a hard-boiled egg are great ways to provide protein. Add some baby carrots with a homemade dip for crunch.

Choose baked over fried. Save the french fries and fried chicken for a special occasion. Try baked sweet potato "fries" or grilled chicken instead.

Choose whole grain over white. Whether you're eating bread, rice, pasta, or even pizza, whole grains will give you more nutrition. In fact, more and more school cafeterias are switching to brown rice and whole-grain bread.

Try leftovers. Was last night's spinach pie, pork roast, or rice and beans a big hit? Make a little extra for lunch.

Take a pass on sugary drinks, such as sweetened fruit drinks or punches. Water and plain low-fat milk are the best drink choices around. Have a kid who won't drink milk? Try making a very light chocolate milk, with a tiny squeeze of chocolate syrup, or mix ¼ cup chocolate milk with ¾ cup plain skim milk.

If your child is buying lunch, review the most healthy choices on the menu with him or her the night before or in the morning. When you're eating out, look at all your options before you place your order.

Dessert is not necessary every day. Many families save dessert for the weekends. And it doesn't need to be a part of lunch. If you think your school has more appealing choices for dessert than for entrées and vegetables, talk to other parents and to your school's cafeteria manager and the school district.

What you eat at home influences what you eat out. If you eat salads at home, your child may be more likely to try the salad bar at school. The good habits you teach your children now can last a lifetime.

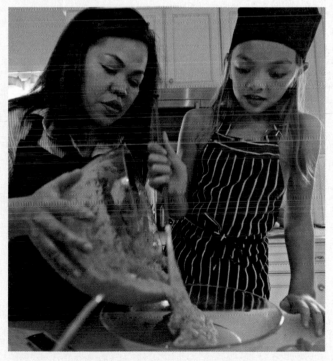

Chef Cris Comerford and her daughter, Danielle.

Ensuring That Every Community Has Access to Healthy, Affordable Food

We know that families living in neighborhoods with a grocery store nearby are more likely to put fresh fruits and vegetables on the table. But every day, 23.5 million Americans, including 6.5 million children, wake up in communities without that basic access to nutritious, affordable food. So we can talk all we want about making healthy choices and serving balanced meals, but that doesn't mean much if parents have no way to access the food they need to actually make those choices and prepare those meals.

Fortunately in recent years, individuals and organizations in every corner of our country have been coming together with one simple mission: to bring fresh food into all our communities. Some have started community gardens. Others are working to attract fresh food retailers. For example, in 2004, the state of Pennsylvania started the Fresh Food Financing Initiative—a partnership among government, businesses, nonprofits, and communities—to help bring supermarkets to underserved areas.

Back then, Philadelphia had fewer supermarkets per person than almost

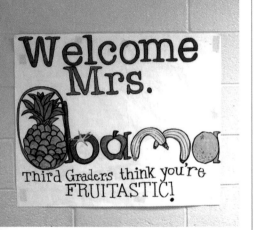

EMBRACING FRESH FOOD IN PHILADELPHIA

In 2010, I visited a brand-new Fresh Grocer in Philadelphia's Progress Plaza. For nearly a decade, there hadn't been a single grocery store in this community. Today, this store is thriving, drawing customers from across the community—and neighboring communities—and turning a profit.

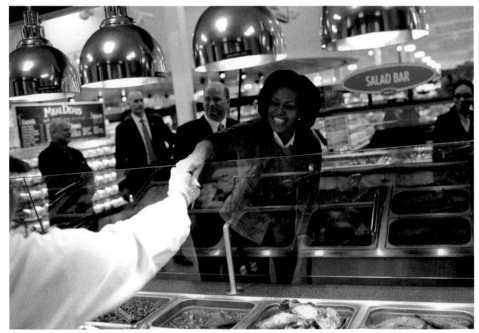

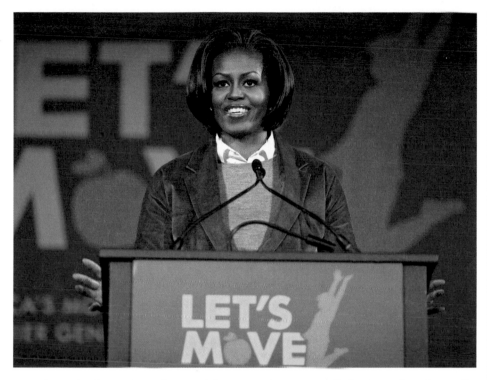

anywhere in America, along with staggering rates of obesity-related conditions like diabetes and heart disease. Since 2004, the Fresh Food Financing Initiative has built more than eighty stores in Pennsylvania, giving more than four hundred thousand people access to nutritious food and creating or preserving five thousand jobs. Philadelphia's efforts have been such a success that we're now trying to do something similar on a national level. In February 2010, as part of *Let's Move!*, we announced the Healthy Food Financing Initiative—a combination of loans, grants, tax credits, and community economic development programs designed to fund new grocery stores, establish farmers' markets, and equip small retailers like corner stores to sell fresh food.

Other communities, including Detroit and Chicago, are reviving the old vegetable truck, a modern-day version of the one that my dad worked on as a boy. Now the trucks are enclosed and refrigerated to keep vegetables and fruits fresh; they're a produce aisle on wheels. This new generation of mobile vegetable sellers, with names like Fresh Moves and Peaches and Greens, visits neighborhoods a couple of times a week, and they do a brisk business.

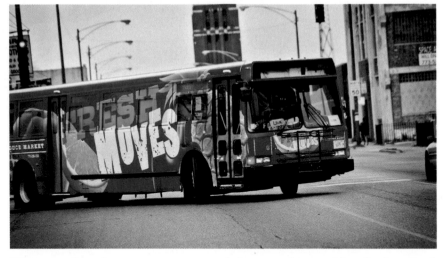

"Our very first day, we were out there on a city street in this big red bus painted with giant fruits and vegetables on the side, and a fourteen-year-old walked by us and asked, 'What is this?' We explained what we do and asked him to pick any piece of fruit that he wanted. Every day, I wish I could replicate the look of joy on his face as he tasted his first organic apple—it was that powerful. He was on his way to play basketball, and we stood there and watched him play basketball with one hand while he held the apple in the other, until it was completely eaten.

"I started Fresh Moves with my partners, Sheelah Muhammad and Jeff Pinzino, after we heard that six hundred thousand people in Chicago were living in under-served areas, without access to fresh fruits and vegetables. Six hundred thousand is a number you can't just walk away from. We started thinking about the way the world used to be, when everything from milk to diapers to heating oil was delivered, and we thought, why not start delivering fresh produce to the people who need it most?

"We looked into mobile homes, RVs, and school buses, but we knew that we needed something that could handle Chicago's weather, where it can break 100 degrees in the summer and be below zero with mounds of snow in the winter. When we learned that by law all Chicago city buses had to be retired every twelve years, we found our answer. We asked the Chicago Transit Authority to give us a bus; and they green-lighted our request in less than five minutes. When it's 25 degrees outside, it's 68 degrees on the bus; when it's 107 degrees outside, it's 68 degrees on the bus, and all our produce stays cool and fresh.

"Our prices are lower than in grocery stores, and many of our products are organic. We get some of our food locally, but Chicago doesn't have a robust growing season, so we also rely on other sources, including parts of the farming community in the South. Our suppliers have lowered their wholesale prices to us and extended us credit. They don't have to do it, but they want to help us serve our community.

"Fresh Moves partners with churches, senior centers, and hospitals all over Chicago's West Side to host stops in neighborhoods without grocery stores. But some of our most popular stops are at schools. We have kids who are coming out to buy fruits and vegetables with their own money; teachers are offering Fresh Moves coupons as rewards for kids who do well in class. And we've become a great school meeting point for parents, who come once a week to the bus.

"Seniors tell us we've revived their shopping experience of fifty years ago. The way the grocery store used to be the hub of communication, that's what's happening on the bus. And today, people from other cities in the United States and from

Canada and Brazil are coming to us to ask how they can start a Fresh Moves program where they live.

"The bus is truly a not-for-profit. All of us still work at our day jobs, but we reached five thousand people in our first six months, sold $30,000 worth of produce, and the cost of the average purchase was about $6.60. Like the ice cream truck, people now expect us to come to their neighborhoods, and if we're late or held up, they start calling, 'Where is Fresh Moves and the big red bus?'"

—STEVE CASEY,
Board President, Fresh Moves

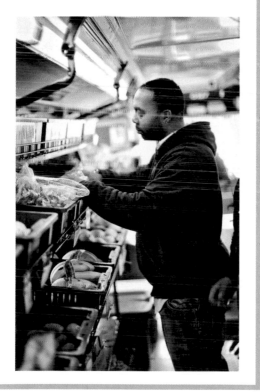

Through *Let's Move!*, we've also been working with corporations across the country to bring more fresh food retailers into our communities. In July 2011, major national chains like SuperValu, Walgreens, and Walmart, as well as regional grocers, committed to building or expanding more than fifteen hundred stores to provide fresh food in underserved areas. The Fresh Works Fund—a coalition of companies and organizations including the California Endowment—agreed to dedicate $200 million to support these efforts in California.

When these stores succeed, they don't just improve our families' health, they can also serve as anchors in our communities, creating jobs and attracting other new businesses to set up shop. All of that can mean even more new jobs and more new customers, which is good for business and good for our communities as well.

But these executives and store owners are making these investments not just as businessmen and -women who care about their companies' bottom lines. They're also doing it as parents and grandparents who care about our kids' health. And they're doing it as leaders who care about our country's future. As Jeffrey Brown, a grocer in Philadelphia, put it, "We're not going to be on the sidelines. We're going to be right with our communities . . . using what we're good at . . . solving problems through innovation and entrepreneurial thinking."

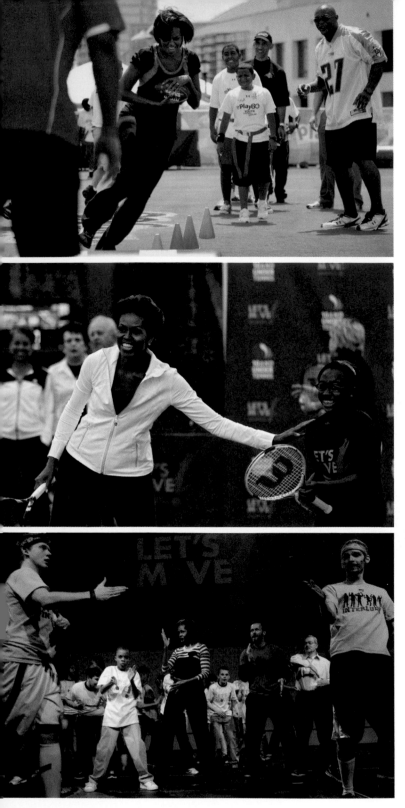

Helping Our Kids Get Moving . . . Literally

Changing the way our kids eat is critical, but it's not enough. We all know that the problem isn't just what's happening at mealtime or snack time. It's also about how our kids are spending the rest of their time each day. It's about how active they are—how much time they spend running around and playing.

Unfortunately, only half of our young people have playgrounds, parks, activity centers, walking paths, or sidewalks in their neighborhoods. Instead of running around outside, kids today are spending an average of 7.5 hours a day in front of some kind of screen. And today fewer than 4 percent of elementary schools, fewer than 8 percent of middle and junior high schools, and only about 2 percent of high schools offer daily PE classes.

Kids' bodies simply are not built for this kind of sedentary lifestyle. They need regular physical activity to build healthy bones and muscles, maintain healthy blood pressure and cholesterol, and control anxiety and stress. That's why *Let's Move!* isn't just about changing how our kids eat—it's about getting them up and moving, literally.

We're working with sports leagues ranging from Major League Baseball to the NFL to encourage kids to get active. We've launched *Let's Move! Outside* to make it easier for kids and families to take advantage of America's beautiful national parks. And we're working with mayors in cities and towns of all sizes who are refurbishing parks and playgrounds, repaving sidewalks and bike paths, and coming up with all kinds of creative ways to get our kids moving.

Playful City, U.S.A., DAVENPORT, IOWA

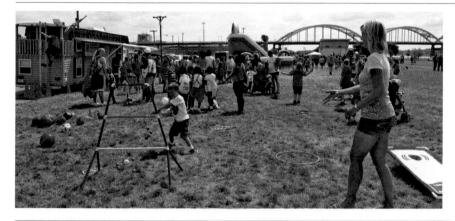

Can a city find new ways for its kids to play? Yes, says Mayor Bill Gulba.

"I hadn't gone to the U.S. Conference of Mayors expecting a challenge from the First Lady about childhood obesity. But I still clearly remember listening to Michelle Obama as she said to all of us, 'We need your help.' I heard the challenge and that's what I wanted to do.

"We had parks in the city that weren't being used, and people were nervous about letting their kids play in them. We wanted to change that, so we took a decommissioned fire truck and stocked it with play equipment: basketballs, tennis equipment, kickballs, soccer balls—and drove it through our parks. We also brought in members of the Community Policing Department to patrol the parks. Sometimes all we had to do was trim the overgrown bushes that were obscuring parks, so people could actually see them and realize that they're safe places to play.

"We've made other changes too, like putting in bike racks at our schools so that kids can ride to school. We're encouraging residents to buy more locally grown food in Davenport, which shouldn't be a heavy lift since the Freight House Farmers' Market operates year-round in our downtown, and there's farmland just ten miles outside our city limits. We're also trying to get healthier foods into our schools and our day care centers so kids can start eating healthier early.

"Our biggest struggle is getting people to stay this course. It's like car makers putting in seat belts. Today it's automatic, but for years such basic safety measures weren't. I'd like us to be one of the healthiest, most active cities in the country. I'd like to keep up my end of the challenge."

—MAYOR BILL GULBA

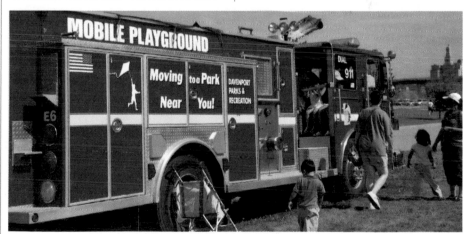

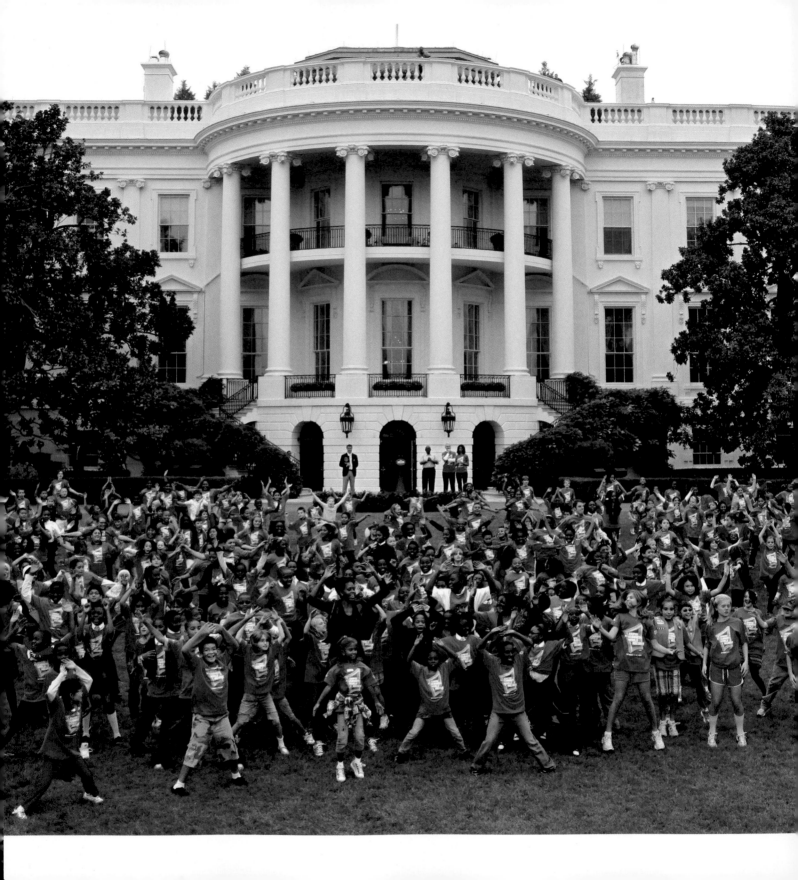

I've hula-hooped and done push-ups on the White House lawn. I've jumped Double Dutch and run through an obstacle course of cardboard boxes carrying water jugs. I've potato-sack raced with comedian Jimmy Fallon. I've even danced "the Dougie" to Beyoncé with a bunch of middle schoolers. But there's a method to my madness. We know that as parents, we are our kids' first and best role models, and I want kids to see that there are all kinds of ways to be active. I also want them to see that being active can be fun—and I'm pretty much willing to make a complete fool of myself if that's what it takes.

That's why, when the weather is nice, we open up the South Lawn for all kinds of sports and fitness activities. In the spring of 2011, when we heard that mega-marathoner Dean Karnazes was passing through Washington, D.C., as part of his run across the country—a journey of three thousand miles to inspire kids and adults to get moving—we decided to invite him to stop by the White House.

On May 2, 2011, Dean, accompanied by TV talk show star Kelly Ripa and three hundred kids from Strong John Thomson and John W. Ross elementary schools in D.C. who had joined him for the last mile and a half of his run, came jogging through the White House gates. Before I knew it, three hundred screaming children were sprinting my way. Praying that I wouldn't be overrun, I opened my arms and cheered them on, giving dozens of hugs and high fives. I made sure to tell them how proud I was of them for being active and showing everyone in D.C. and across the nation just how easy it is to get moving.

Several months later, in the fall of 2011, we worked with *National Geographic Kids* to invite more than four hundred kids to do jumping jacks on the South Lawn in the hopes of breaking the old Guinness World Record for most people doing jumping jacks in a twenty-four-hour period. The number to beat was 20,454. We had intended to have the kids jumping in rows, but kids doing jumping jacks don't necessarily stay in neat lines. Pretty soon, it was one big jumping-jack mass with arms and legs flying in every direction. But we helped break the record—Guinness World Record officials have certified that an incredible 300,265 people across America and around the world jumped that day. The kids learned how much fun it is to get active, and I was reminded once again how every time we open up the South Lawn for activities or for visits to the garden, it helps make the White House everybody's home.

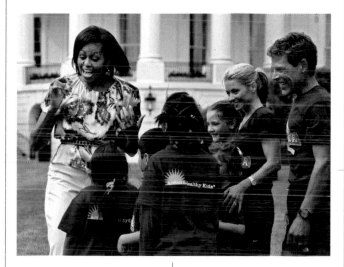

BREAKING THE GUINNESS WORLD RECORD
It took a lot of jumping, but on October 11, 2011, on the White House South Lawn, we helped break the World Record for most people doing jumping jacks in a 24-hour period (opposite).

A LITTLE ENCOURAGEMENT
As part of mega-marathoner Dean Karnazes' 2011 run across America, Dean and TV talk show star Kelly Ripa show kids from Washington, D.C., how easy it is to get moving (above).

Good Role Models for Getting Active

The President's Council on Fitness, Sports & Nutrition is a committee of high-profile volunteers whose mission is to educate, inspire, and empower all Americans to adopt a healthy lifestyle that includes regular physical activity and good nutrition. Council members like Dominique Dawes, Grant Hill, and Michelle Kwan serve as important role models, encouraging young people to get—and stay—active.

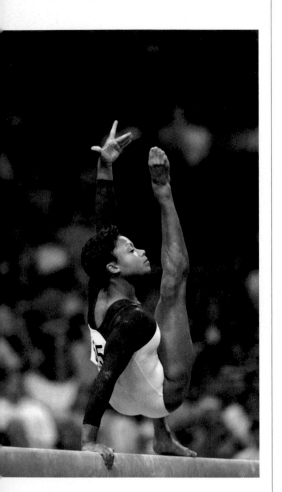

"When I was young, I didn't always want to wake up at five a.m., train from six to eight a.m., then go to school and head back to the gym to train more at night. But I had a fabulous coach, Kelli Hill, who motivated me, and I had my teammates. I loved the camaraderie—I wouldn't quit on them, and they wouldn't quit on me. To keep fit, it's important to find that same kind of motivation, whether it's from the company you keep or from within yourself. Working out or being active each day gives me mental clarity and stabilizes my mood. When I'm exercising, I notice that people enjoy being around me more.

"I also need to eat well. Eating a diet low in nutrients catches up with me after a couple of days. I'm not necessarily a healthy eater all the time, but I'm very good about moderation. You don't have to totally nix certain less healthy foods from your diet—just eat them rarely, and don't eat a huge portion. Small steps like this make a huge difference. That applies to physical activity as well. If you're blessed with the ability to move your legs, try parking farther away in a parking lot. Walk your dog. At work, take the stairs rather than the elevator or escalator. Walk the stairs in your house during TV commercials. Even the smallest changes can add up over time."

—Dominique Dawes,
co-chair of the President's Council on Fitness, Sports & Nutrition,
and three-time Olympian and gold medalist in gymnastics

"Even a pro athlete isn't motivated to exercise or train all the time. When I am not motivated, the first thing I concentrate on is shifting my mind-set. I like to think of how my previous trips to the gym have helped me achieve success. I also try to think of a reward to give myself post-workout, something like drinking a fruit smoothie, or eating fresh fruit, or reading a new book. And I know how important it is to eat healthy and stay active, not just to succeed in sports, but also to succeed in life. I like to eat a lot of fruits and vegetables, and for the most part, I only drink water. When I eat healthy, stay hydrated, and am active, I have a clearer mind to help me accomplish my goals on and off the court, as a professional athlete and as a husband and father."

— Grant Hill,

professional basketball player, Phoenix Suns,
winner of the NBA Rookie of the Year award
and now the second-oldest player in the NBA

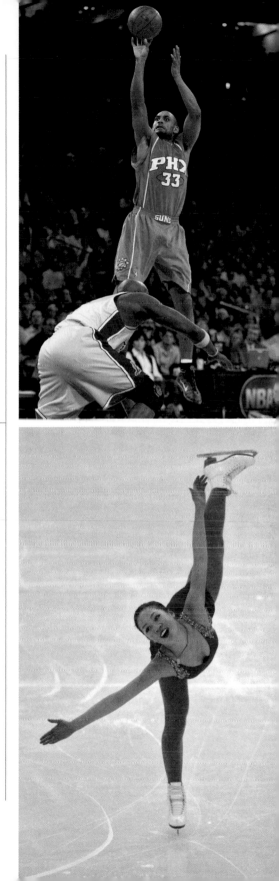

"Not every athlete eats healthy. I started off eating junk food, candy bars, and ice cream. But when I was fifteen, I started paying attention to what my role models were eating. They all chose a healthy diet, and I mimicked what they ate. I saw huge results in my skating. Eating well is such a key element of performing well. When I improved my diet, I could focus for a lot longer. Twenty-five minutes had been my max. After I changed my habits, I could go for hours. Even now that I'm not training for the Olympics, I still have to eat healthy—if I don't, I can really feel it. I've found that little things really add up, like having a salad every day with light dressing and eating fruit. I know how hard it is to stay active. But if you can walk, swim, go to the park, or play outside, it becomes a lifestyle. And it can make a lifelong difference."

—Michelle Kwan,

two-time Olympic medalist,
and the most decorated figure skater in U.S. history

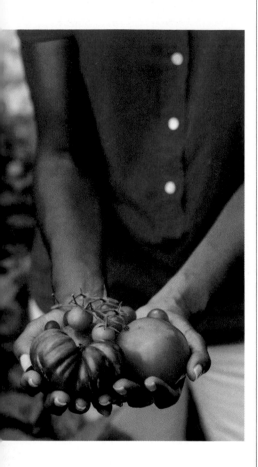

Growing Momentum

Every day, we're seeing more and more people across this country coming together on behalf of our children's health. Nearly five hundred museums, gardens, and zoos have signed up to offer active exhibits and healthy food choices. The United States Tennis Association has built or refurbished thousands of kid-friendly tennis courts—the courts are smaller, the nets are lower, and the balls used are bigger. Faith and community organizations have literally stepped up and walked more than 2.8 million miles, and they're sponsoring summer nutrition programs for kids and exercise ministries for families. And for the first time in twenty years, the military is improving the food they serve to our service members and their families on bases and in facilities across the country.

Kids themselves are taking action as well. In November 2010, I met a little boy in Newark, New Jersey, who had been paying attention when his teacher did a unit on healthy eating. That night, when he got home, he insisted that his mother bake rather than fry the fish she was cooking for dinner. And a little girl wrote me a letter to let me know that when she saw a public service announcement for *Let's Move!*, she and her friend put down the junk food they were eating and went for a bike ride.

Most important of all, parents are getting involved, serving healthier food at home and helping their kids get—and stay—active. They're making a difference in our schools, workplaces, and communities too. For example, when Aaron Marks, a father from Decatur, Georgia, found out that his four-year-old son was eating pizza for breakfast at school and doughnuts and cookies for snacks, he talked to the school's administrators. He also joined the school's nutrition committee and helped raise money to plant a garden. As he put it, "You can't just take no for an answer. You have to be tenacious."

You wouldn't necessarily expect such a diverse collection of individuals and organizations to all be working on the same issue. But we are drawn together by our shared commitment to our children's future. We all want so much for our children. We want them to succeed at everything they do. We want to protect them from every hardship and spare them from every mistake. But we know we can't do all of that. What we can do, however, is give them the very best start in their journeys. Together we can give them advantages early in life that will stay with them long after we're gone. As President Franklin Roosevelt once put it, "We cannot always build the future for our youth, but we can build our youth for the future."

That is precisely what we are doing. And while we still have a long way to go, every day, with passion and imagination, we are coming up with new ideas and solutions. Every day, with steps large and small, we are getting closer to our goal of giving all our kids the healthy future they deserve.

And it all started with a garden.

NEW BEGINNINGS
On our first planting day back in 2009, I could never have imagined all the wonderful ideas and initiatives that would start to grow from our White House Kitchen Garden.

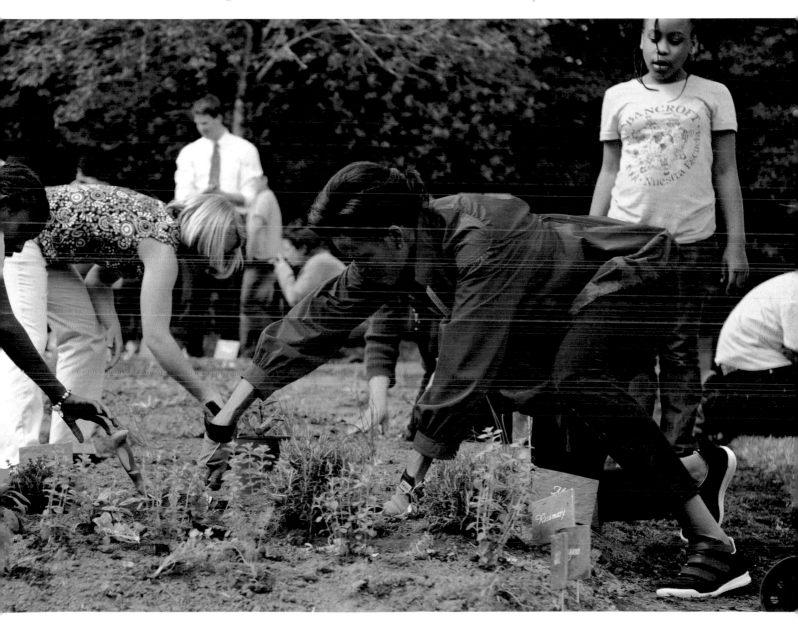

THE 2011
Winter Garden
PLAN

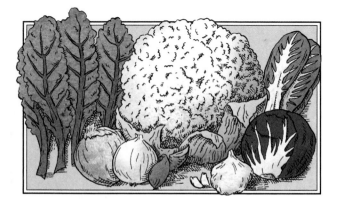

"In a garden, with a little ingenuity and imagination—and a whole lot of effort—you can achieve something you never thought possible."

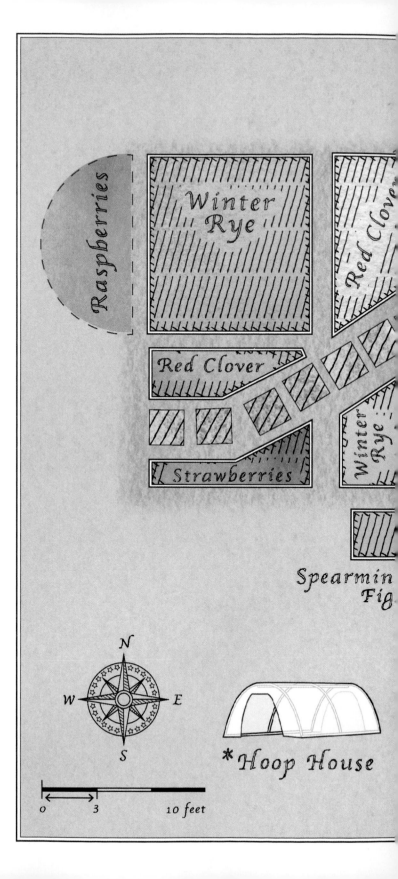

Raspberries

Winter Rye

Red Clover

Red Clover

Winter Rye

Strawberries

Spearmint
Fig

N
W   E
S

*Hoop House

0   3   10 feet

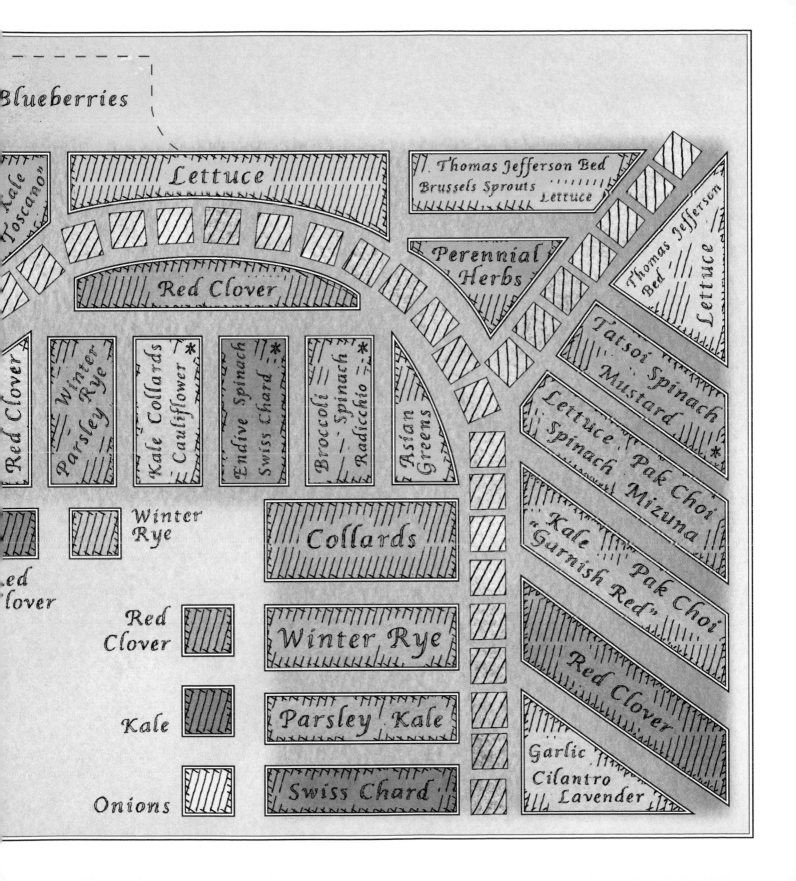

Blueberries

Kale "Toscano"

Lettuce

Thomas Jefferson Bed
Brussels Sprouts
Lettuce

Thomas Jefferson Bed

Thomas Jefferson Lettuce

Red Clover

Perennial Herbs

Red Clover

Winter Rye
Parsley

Kale Collards
Cauliflower *

Endive Spinach
Swiss Chard *

Broccoli
Spinach
Radicchio *

Asian Greens

Tatsoi Spinach
Mustard

Lettuce Pak Choi
Spinach Mizuna

Kale "Garnish Red"
Pak Choi

Winter Rye

Collards

Red Clover

Red Clover

Winter Rye

Kale

Parsley Kale

Garlic
Cilantro
Lavender

Onions

Swiss Chard

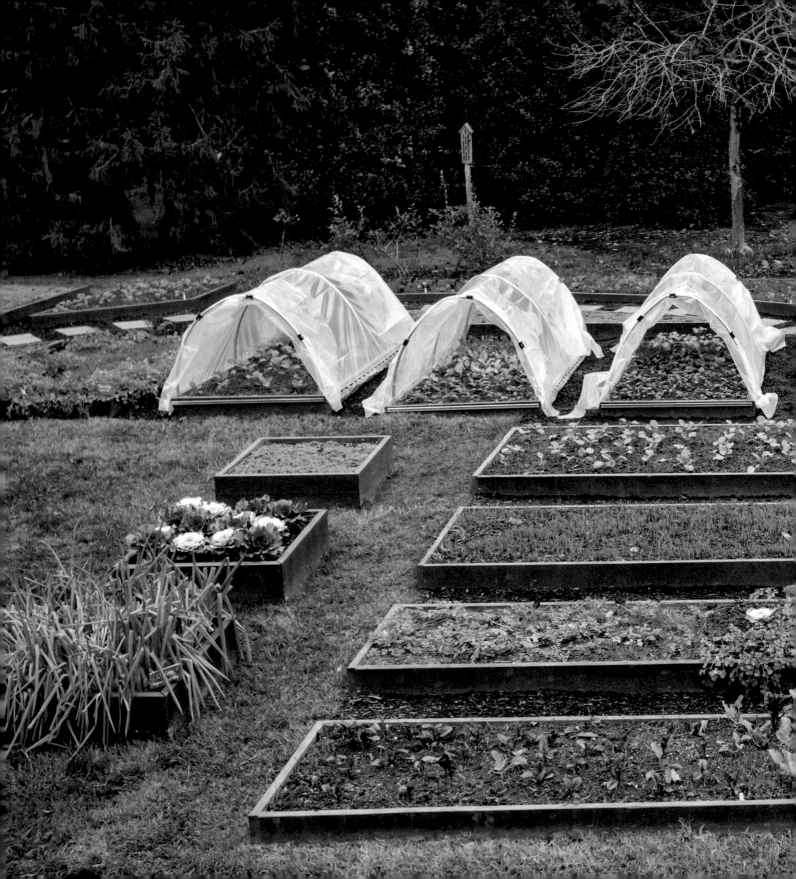

THE WINTER GARDEN 2011

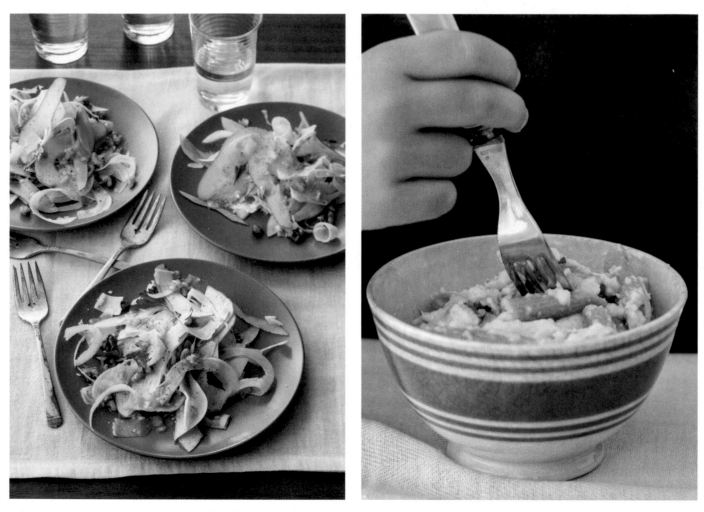

winter salad
page 251

cauliflower mac and cheese
page 252

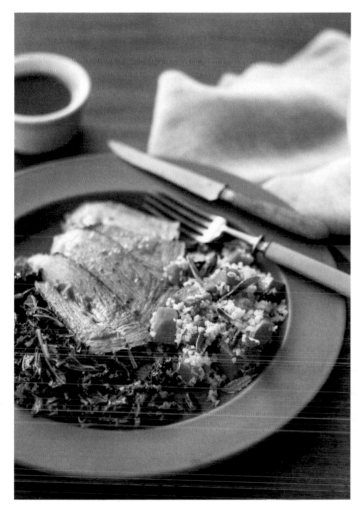

braised pork shoulder with
butternut squash and greens
page 255

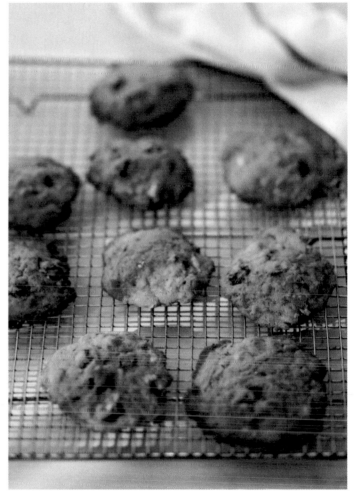

white chocolate–cherry–carrot
cookies
page 258

That first winter in the garden, I was reminded that with creativity, commitment, and hard work, we can overcome even the most seemingly insurmountable obstacles. Every day, individuals and communities across our country are bringing that lesson to life on behalf of our children. They remind me of those little plants that thrive in the harshest conditions, succeeding against all odds to help our children lead healthier lives. Their stories fill me with hope about our future.

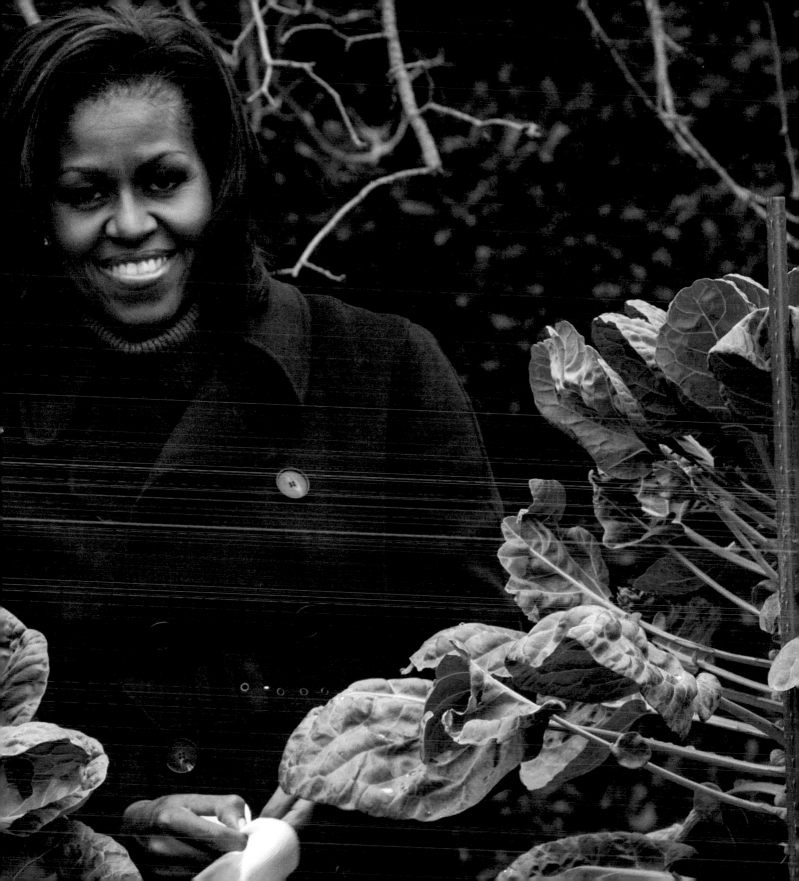

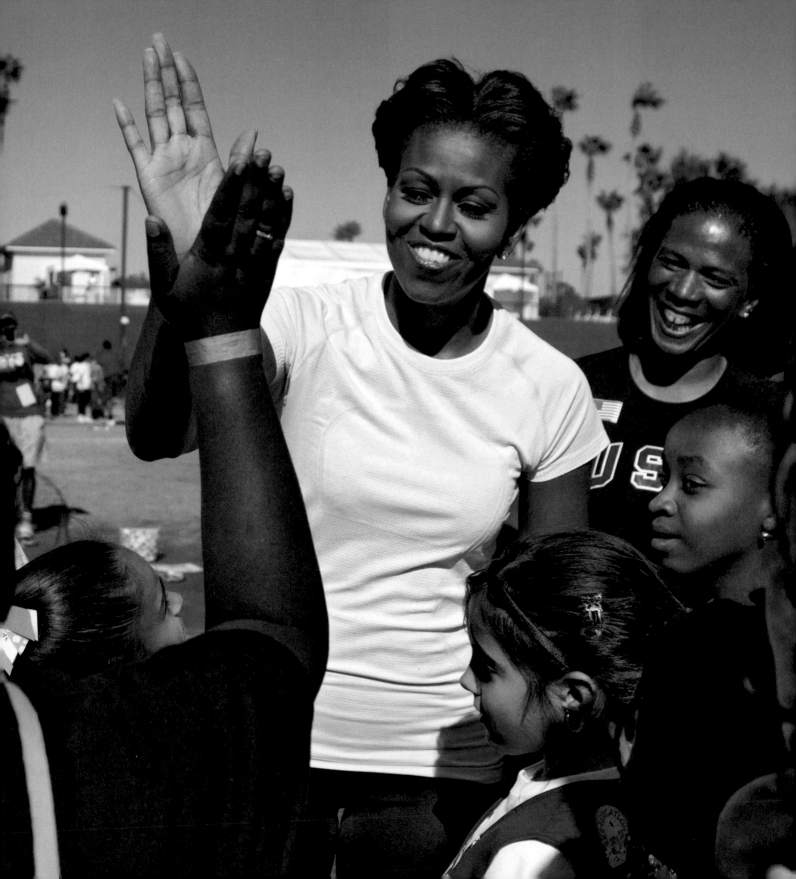

CONCLUSION:
THE SEEDS WE HAVE PLANTED

Every week, I get letters from kids and from schools asking about our garden and telling us about their own gardens and their own efforts to eat healthily. It makes me especially happy to receive letters like the one I received from the Avoyelles Public Charter School, which read, "We are inspired by your examples of planting a garden at the White House and encouraging children to eat healthy and exercise. Here in Mansura, Louisiana—against all odds with no budget—we started an Edible Schoolyard." Enclosed were pictures of the kids, one with a handwritten caption that read, "It all starts with a seed."

That, more than anything, is the message I hope to convey with this book. So often, gardens start with so little—a few neighbors who want to reclaim an empty plot, a family that wants to put healthier meals on the table, a school that wants to teach kids how their food is grown. But the impact our gardens have on our lives—and the life of our nation—is anything but small. Whether it's a few plants in the backyard or on the windowsill, a small garden near the town center, or a vast tract of land with crops as far as the eye can see, year after year, season after season, gardens bring individuals and communities together. They provide fresh, nutritious food for our families. They inspire and engage our children, teaching them

TIME TO CELEBRATE
Celebrating the second anniversary of Let's Move! *with kids and Paralympian April Holmes at the ESPN Wide World of Sports Complex at Walt Disney World.*

the value of hard work and teamwork and showing them just how delicious food can taste when it's fresh from the vine.

For me, planting a garden was a way to help start a national conversation about the health of our children, an issue I care deeply about, not just as First Lady but as a mother. It's an issue I often think about as my family sits down for dinner. Barack, Malia, Sasha, and I eat together pretty much every night at 6:30 p.m.; even if Barack is traveling, he always tries to make it back home in time for dinner. We start our meal by saying grace—and our grace always ends with "We hope we live long and strong"—and we talk with our daughters about what's going on in their lives, and in ours. Some nights, we discuss issues they've heard about in the news. Other nights, we talk through situations they've encountered in the classroom or on the playground, and we strategize about how to navigate the complicated world of elementary and middle school friendships. Many nights, as I look at my children, I think of my hopes for them—and for all our children: that they grow up healthy; that they have the energy, strength, and stamina to build families and careers of

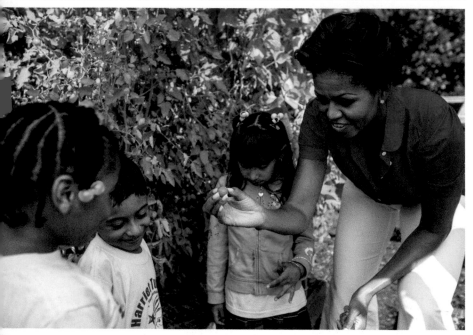

their own; that they can pursue every last one of their dreams and fulfill every last bit of their potential.

Whether it's sitting down for that family dinner, growing a tomato out on the stoop, or just taking our kids for a walk in the park, we all have a role to play in building this future for our children. Each of us has the opportunity—and the responsibility—to begin planting those seeds in our families and communities. And on behalf of our children, I hope that each of us, in our own way, will take up this charge.

Michelle Obama

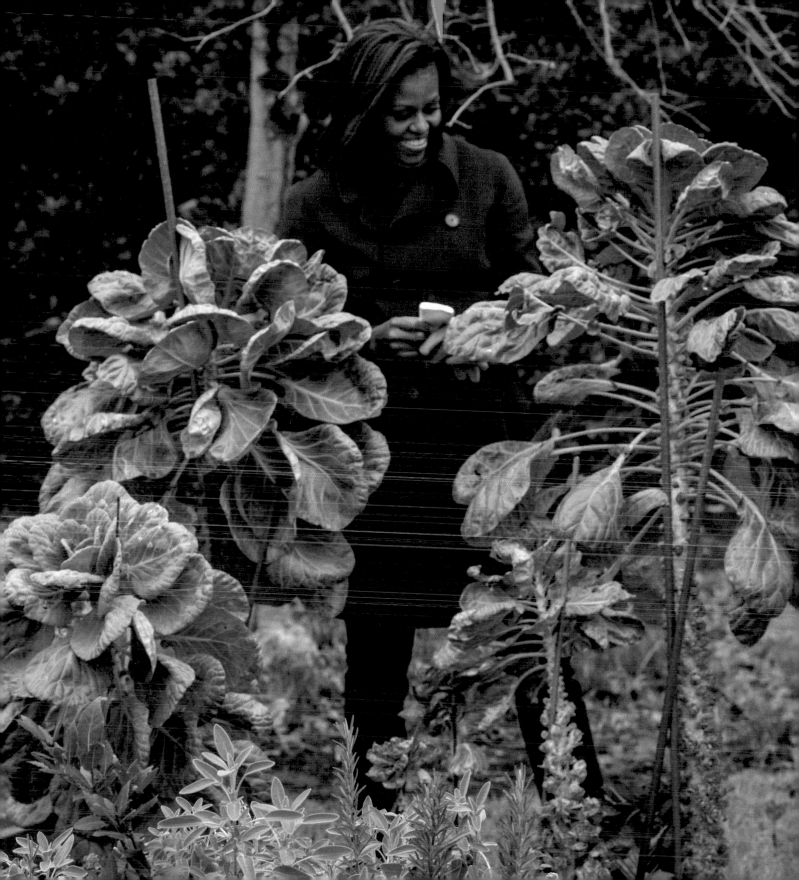

Garden Highlights & Recipes

SPRING GARDEN HIGHLIGHTS
Tips from Executive Chef Cris Comerford

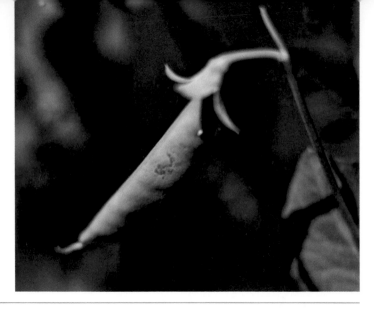

Peas: Peas are rich in protein and fiber. Use a minimal amount of water when cooking fresh or frozen peas to help preserve their vitamin C. Frozen peas are a great choice all year round, but fresh peas have a unique flavor. Select pods that are firm, velvety, and smooth, with a bright, medium green color. Avoid puffy pods or any that have a rattling sound; fresh peas are tightly packed. Fresh peas should be stored in the refrigerator and will keep for several days.

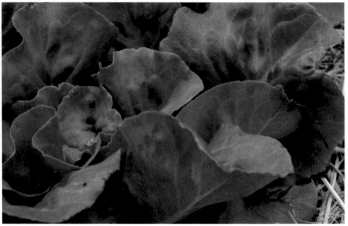

Lettuce: Darker-colored lettuces have more nutrients. Look for lettuce with no signs of wilting, slimy leaves, or spots. Lettuce needs refrigeration to stay fresh and keeps well in airtight plastic bags. Iceberg lasts the longest at up to two weeks. Romaine will keep for up to ten days; butterheads keep four to five days. Loose greens should be eaten sooner. When washing greens, do not rip them into smaller pieces before you run them under the water because the leaves will lose their nutrients. Instead cut or tear them after you dry them.

Rhubarb and Strawberries: Strawberries have one of the lowest sugar contents of all fruits. Rhubarb is also low in sugar, and it's high in calcium and vitamins. When selecting rhubarb, choose fresh, crisp stalks. Peel off any fibrous strings, and cut off any leaves (which are poisonous) as well as the ends of the stalk. With the leaves removed, you can store the stalks for up to three weeks in sealed plastic bags before cooking. For strawberries, choose the plumpest, most fragrant berries. Small and medium berries tend to be sweeter and juicier. Strawberries keep best in an open container or colander. Don't wash them until you are ready to use. Most berries should be eaten within one to three days.

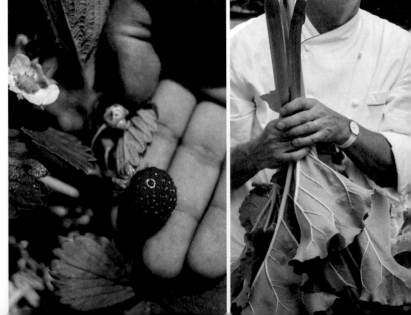

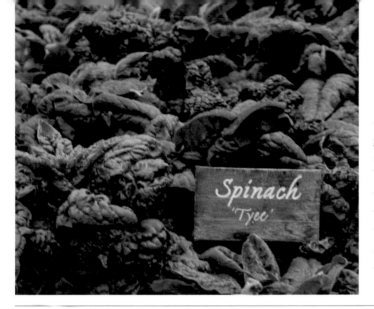

Spinach: Spinach leaves come in two varieties, flat or curly, and can be eaten raw or cooked. Although spinach grows best in Washington, D.C., in the spring or fall, it is available in stores all year round. If you cut the outside leaves of a spinach plant, its inside leaves will continue to grow. Fresh spinach should be lightly dried and stored unwashed in the refrigerator in a sealed plastic bag for three to four days. Make sure you wash fresh spinach several times thoroughly before eating to remove any dirt and grit.

Parsley: Parsley plants will reappear in the garden season after season. Parsley is best stored in the refrigerator, where it can keep for up to twenty-one days. Wash and drain it and then keep it in a sealed container or a bag with a paper towel or cloth underneath to help control moisture.

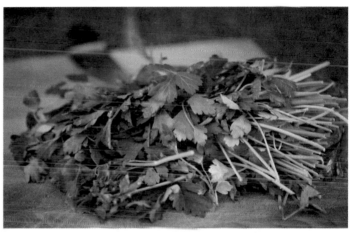

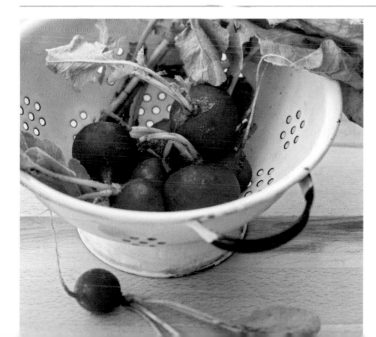

Radishes: Most Americans eat radishes raw in salads, but they can also be cooked, and they can serve as a substitute for turnips in some recipes. Choose firm radishes with good color and no cracks. Remove any green tops before storing because the tops will siphon moisture and nutrients from the radishes. Radishes keep best wrapped in a moist towel and stored in a plastic container in the coldest part of the refrigerator, where they can remain fresh for at least a week.

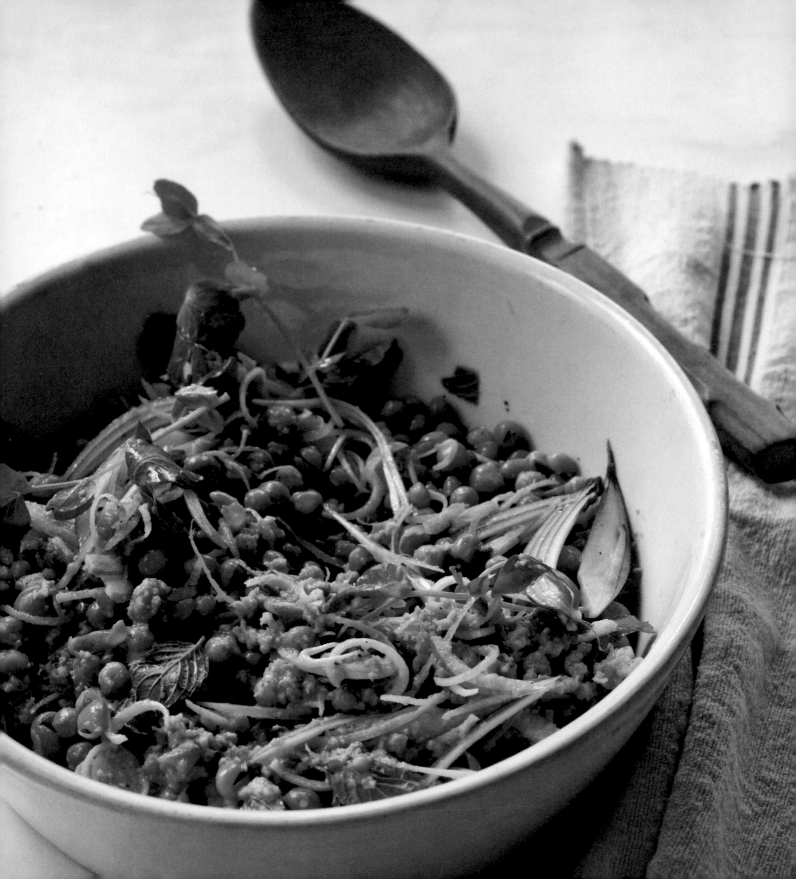

spring pea salad

SERVES 6 TO 8

Sweet green peas, fresh from the garden or the farmers' market, are so delicious that you don't need to hide their bright color or delicate flavor underneath heavy dressings or a lot of butter. In this recipe, the peas are enhanced by a dressing made with pureed peas, mint, and the citrusy smell and taste of lemon to welcome the spring. —CHEF CRIS

1. Bring a large pot of salted water to a boil. Pour the peas into the water and cook for no more than 2 minutes. Drain and immediately plunge the peas into a bowl of ice water. Drain and pat dry with a towel. Puree ½ cup of the peas in a blender.

2. Place the peas, pea puree, shallot, and leek in a medium glass or stainless steel bowl and toss gently to combine.

3. Add the lemon zest and juice, olive oil, and mint. Season with salt and pepper and toss gently until the vegetables are coated. Serve immediately.

2½ cups shelled fresh green peas
1 small shallot, thinly sliced
1 small leek (white part only), cleaned and thinly sliced
Zest and juice of 1 lemon
¼ cup extra-virgin olive oil
½ cup shredded fresh mint leaves
Salt and freshly ground black pepper

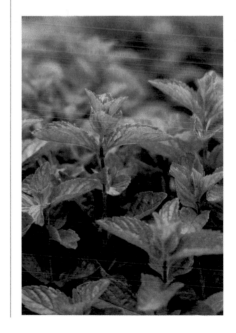

spinach pie

SERVES 6 TO 8

Fresh spinach takes a starring role in this satisfying, savory pie. Perfect for a busy family, it can be made in advance and served hot, cold, or at room temperature. Try it for lunch, brunch, or dinner, served with a light green salad and fruit for dessert. I like to put a dollop of Greek yogurt on my portion for extra tartness.

You can use whole or 2% milk instead of half-and-half if you prefer.

—CHEF CRIS

1 9-inch unbaked piecrust
2 tablespoons olive oil
6 cloves garlic, minced
1 small onion, chopped
1 pound fresh spinach, well washed and drained
Salt and freshly ground black pepper
2 large eggs, beaten
1 cup half-and-half
1 teaspoon grated lemon zest
1 teaspoon chopped fresh thyme leaves
6 ounces feta cheese, crumbled
8 ounces Swiss cheese, grated

1. Preheat the oven to 375 degrees F. Place the piecrust on a rimmed baking sheet lined with foil or parchment paper.

2. In a medium skillet over medium heat, drizzle in the olive oil. Add the garlic and onion and sauté until translucent, 5 to 7 minutes. Do not let the garlic burn. Add the spinach, a little at a time, and cook until wilted. Season with salt and pepper and set aside to cool.

3. In a medium bowl, whisk together the eggs and half-and-half. Add the lemon zest and thyme. Add the spinach, the feta cheese, and half the Swiss cheese and mix until well combined. Season with salt and pepper.

4. Pour the mixture carefully into the piecrust and sprinkle the remaining Swiss cheese evenly over the top.

5. Bake for about 40 minutes, or until the center is set. Cool for at least 10 minutes before serving.

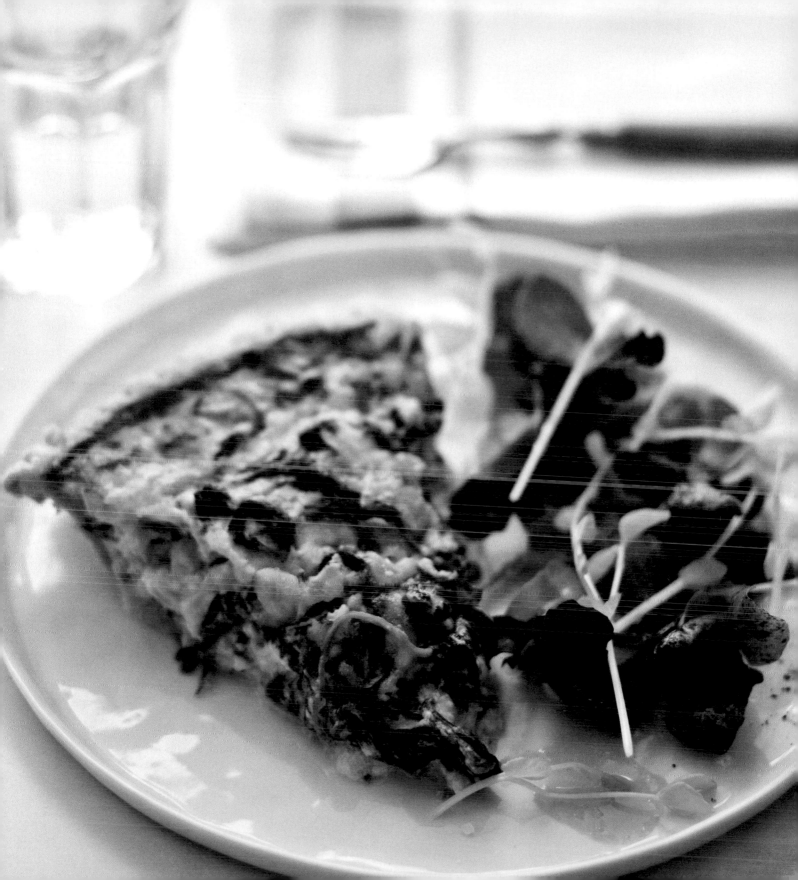

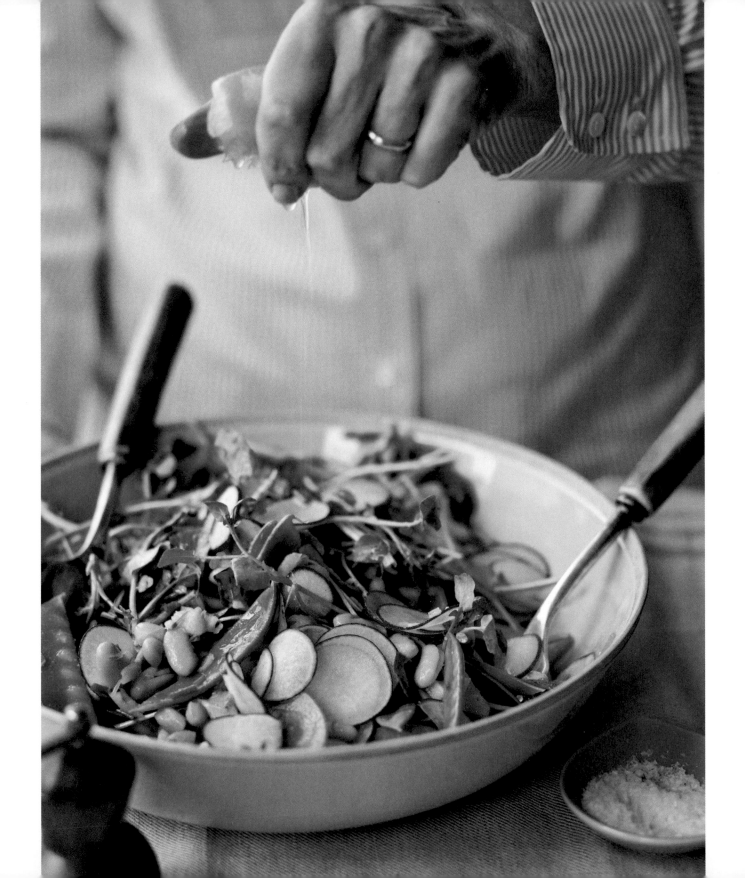

white bean salad

SERVES 6 TO 8 AS A STARTER

Creamy white beans, fresh basil, and crunchy young vegetables are combined in a light but substantial salad that takes advantage of the first fruits of the spring garden. Use a mild honey, like clover or wildflower. —CHEF SAM

1. If you're using dried beans, first rinse them, picking out any stones, and then place them in a bowl. Cover with cold water and soak for 8 hours or overnight, then drain the beans and place in a pot. Add the garlic and bay leaf and enough water to cover the beans by at least 1 inch. Bring to a boil, reduce the heat, cover, and simmer, stirring occasionally, until the beans are tender, about 1 hour.

2. In a small bowl, combine the olive oil, lemon zest, lemon juice, honey, and shallot to make a vinaigrette. Whisk to combine.

3. When the beans are done, drain them well and place in a medium bowl. Discard the bay leaf and garlic clove. Add one third of the vinaigrette to the warm beans and toss; then let stand for 15 minutes, tossing occasionally. If using canned beans, rinse and drain them and then toss with the vinaigrette.

4. In a small pot of boiling water, cook the snow peas for 1 minute. Using a slotted spoon, place them in a bowl of ice water. Drain, pat dry, and thinly slice.

5. In a large salad bowl, place the cooled beans, snow peas, chives, radishes, and basil. Pour the remaining dressing over and toss lightly. Serve immediately.

1 cup dried small white beans, such as cannellini or Great Northern, or 1 15-ounce can
1 clove garlic
1 bay leaf
¼ cup extra-virgin olive oil
½ teaspoon grated lemon zest
1 tablespoon lemon juice
½ teaspoon honey
1 tablespoon chopped shallot
1 cup snow peas or sugar snap peas
½ bunch fresh chives, chopped
5 mild radishes, such as Lady Slipper radishes, thinly sliced
3 tablespoons chopped fresh basil

rhubarb strawberry crumble pie

SERVES 6 TO 8

It is a well-known fact that President Obama loves pie, and in the pastry kitchen we rack our brains trying to create new combinations. This one is pretty classic, but you can replace the strawberries with blackberries, apples, peaches, or nectarines; the tart rhubarb goes well with all of those sweet fruits. —CHEF BILL

FOR THE PIECRUST
(OR USE ONE PREPARED
10-INCH CRUST)
1 cup (2 sticks) unsalted butter,
    cut into small (½-inch) cubes,
    plus additional for greasing the
    pie plate
2½ leveled cups all-purpose flour
1 teaspoon salt
1 teaspoon sugar
5 tablespoons cold water

FOR THE FILLING
4 cups rhubarb, washed,
    trimmed, and cut into 1-inch
    lengths
2 cups fresh strawberries, rinsed,
    patted dry, and hulled
½ cup turbinado* or raw sugar
½ cup honey
1 teaspoon pure vanilla extract
¼ teaspoon salt
6 tablespoons all-purpose flour

1. **Make the crust:** Butter a 10-inch pie plate.

2. Freeze the butter cubes for 10 minutes.

3. In the bowl of an electric mixer, combine the flour, salt, and sugar on low speed. Add the cold butter and mix, using short on-and-off bursts, until the dough has the consistency of coarse cornmeal. If there are a few larger pieces of dough, that's fine.

4. Add the water in a slow stream until the dough forms a ball and then stop mixing. Invert the dough onto a work surface and finish mixing by hand, sprinkling a little more flour on it if necessary. The dough will be mealy and uneven with spots of butter. Push down into a 2-inch-thick disk. Wrap the dough in plastic wrap and refrigerate for at least 2 hours or overnight.

5. Remove the dough from the refrigerator and sprinkle the work surface and a rolling pin with a little flour (about a tablespoon) to prevent sticking. Roll the dough out to a large rectangle and then fold it over on itself like a book. Reroll out to a 14-inch circle ⅛ to ¼ inch thick. Roll the dough onto the rolling pin, center the pin over the pie plate, and gently unroll the dough over the prepared plate. Ease the dough into the bottom of the plate and fit it to the sides; cut away excess with scissors and flute the edges.

6. Place the piecrust in the freezer for about 30 minutes to firm up the dough.

7. **Make the filling**: In a large bowl, gently combine the rhubarb and strawberries. Add the turbinado sugar, honey, vanilla, and salt and toss lightly.

8. Sift the flour over the top, stir in to evenly coat the fruit, and set aside.

9. **Make the topping**: In an electric mixer or food processor, mix the flour, brown sugar, and oats. Add the butter and mix or pulse briefly until clumps form.

10. Position the oven rack in the lower third of the oven. Preheat the oven to 350 degrees F. Remove the piecrust from the freezer.

11. Pour the fruit mixture into the crust and sprinkle evenly with the topping. Place the pie plate on a baking sheet lined with foil or parchment (for easier cleanup) and bake for 1 hour and 10 minutes, or until the pie is bubbling and the crust is golden brown.

FOR THE TOPPING
1 cup all-purpose flour
⅔ cup (packed) light brown sugar
½ cup quick-cooking oats
½ cup (1 stick) unsalted butter, cold and cut into small pieces

Turbinado sugar is a raw sugar that is light brown with larger crystals than granulated sugar. It can be found in the baking section of the supermarket.

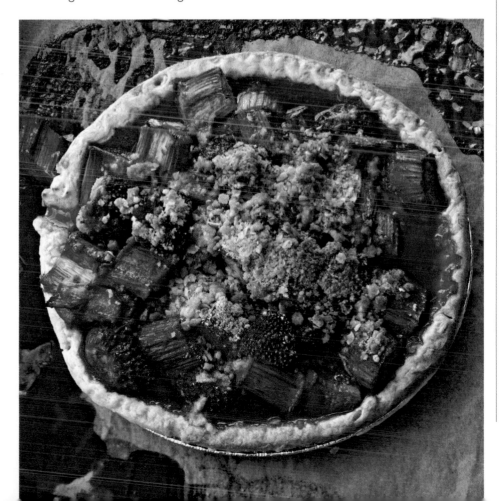

SUMMER GARDEN HIGHLIGHTS
Tips from Executive Chef Cris Comerford

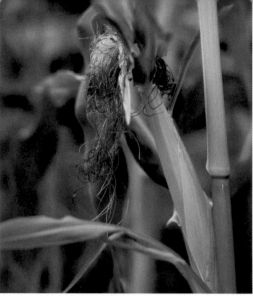

Corn: Corn needs to be stored in a cool environment to protect its natural sugars and is best eaten within one to two days of picking. The husks should be green and have visible kernels that are plump and tightly packed on the cob. The liquid inside the kernels should be light and milky colored. When you bring corn home, refrigerate it immediately.

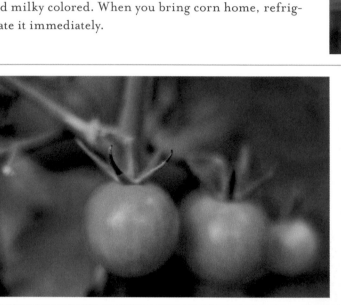

Tomatoes and Basil: Store tomatoes on a counter on their "shoulders," the indented side where the stem was attached, and keep them separated rather than touching. Once ripe, eat within twelve to twenty-four hours; otherwise freeze, cook, or refrigerate to prevent them from rotting. Tomatoes are often paired with basil, which can be kept fresh by keeping the stems in a cup of water as you would flowers. Don't cut basil until just before serving.

Shell Beans: The best way to select green beans is loose rather than prepackaged, so that you can choose the individual beans. Look for beans with a smooth feel and vibrant green color, free from brown spots or bruises. They should be firm and should "snap" when broken. Store the beans unwashed in a plastic bag in the refrigerator crisper, where they may keep for up to seven days.

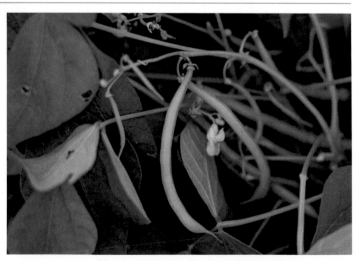

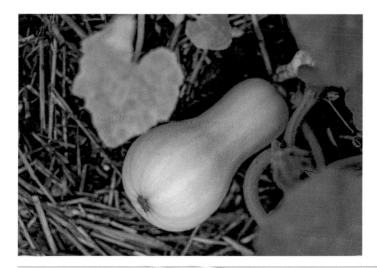

Squash: When selecting squash, look for a heavy feel and shiny, unblemished rinds. The rinds should not be very hard; tough rinds are a sign of overmatured squash. Medium-size squash have the best taste and the softest flesh. Handle carefully because even small rind punctures can cause the vegetable to decay. Store unwashed in the refrigerator in a bag or airtight container for up to seven days.

Blueberries: Every year we try to grow blueberries, and every year the birds get to them before we do. In the summer of 2011, out of the entire bush, two blueberries made it, but Mrs. Obama said they were two of the most delicious blueberries she has ever tasted. When selecting blueberries, look for firm berries with a bright, uniform hue. Berries should not be too tightly packed. If they don't move, that could be an indication of mold or damage.

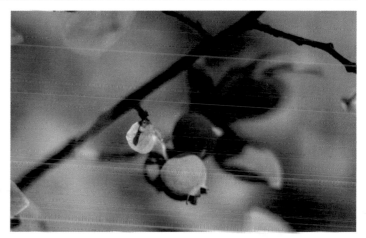

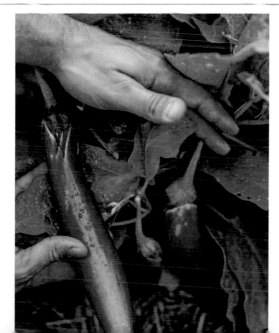

Eggplant: When selecting eggplants, look for ones that are heavy for their size. The color should be bright and vivid and the skin should be firm and free from scars, bruises, or discoloration. A ripe eggplant's skin will spring back from a gentle press of the thumb. Eggplants are highly perishable and are sensitive to extremes of heat or cold. They can ripen on a counter until slightly wrinkly and then should be cooked immediately or refrigerated. Don't force an eggplant into a crisper bin—doing so may damage its skin.

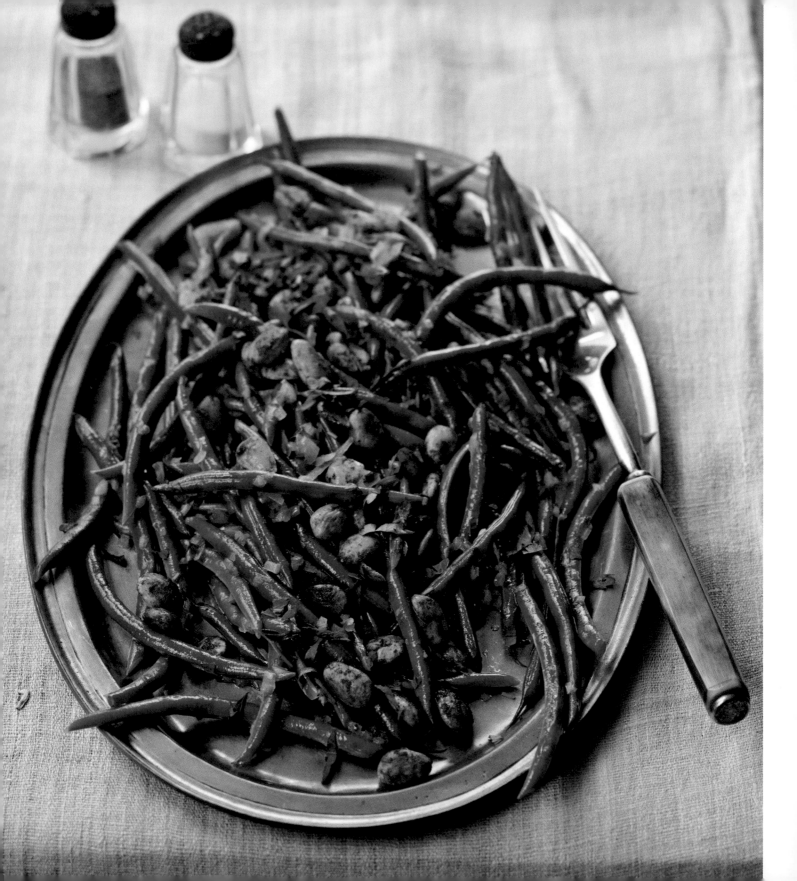

green beans
with almonds

SERVES 6 TO 8

This twist on a classic side dish makes any grilled or roasted poultry or meat special. You can use any kind of almonds that you have on hand. Shallots have a mild, sweet onion flavor, but you can substitute the same amount of regular onions or even leeks or scallions if you prefer. And if you can't find flat-leaf parsley, curly will do as well. —CHEF CRIS

1. Bring a large pot of salted water to a boil. Cook the green beans for about 5 minutes. Drain and place the beans in a large bowl of ice water to cool quickly. Drain again and set aside.

2. Preheat the oven to 350 degrees F. On a rimmed baking sheet lined with foil, toss the almonds with the melted butter and paprika. Spread in a single layer and bake for 7 minutes, or just until fragrant. Do not let the almonds burn. Remove from the oven and set aside.

3. In a medium pan over medium heat, warm the olive oil and butter. Add the shallots and sauté for 2 to 3 minutes. Add the green beans and sauté until warmed through. Remove from the heat and add the parsley. Season with salt and pepper.

4. Place the beans in a serving dish and garnish with the toasted almonds. Serve immediately.

1½ pounds fresh green beans, washed and trimmed
1 cup slivered almonds
1 teaspoon melted butter
1 teaspoon sweet paprika
1 teaspoon extra-virgin olive oil
1 tablespoon butter
2 shallots, minced (about ¼ cup)
1 tablespoon chopped fresh flat-leaf parsley
Salt and freshly ground black pepper

FOR THE SALAD

1 cup fresh corn kernels

Salt and freshly ground black pepper

½ pound green beans, trimmed

1 pound assorted summer lettuces, such as Bibb, romaine, and red leaf, well washed and dried

½ cucumber, peeled and cut into ½-inch cubes

2 mild radishes, such as breakfast radishes, trimmed and thinly sliced

1 ripe tomato, cut into ½-inch cubes

½ bell pepper, cut into ½-inch cubes

3 to 4 scallions (white part only), chopped

FOR THE PECANS

½ cup pecan halves

1 tablespoon honey

1½ teaspoons brown sugar

1½ teaspoons melted unsalted butter

½ teaspoon Cajun spice mixture

FOR THE DRESSING

¼ cup white wine vinegar

Juice of 1 lemon

1 shallot, minced (about 1 tablespoon)

1 tablespoon chopped fresh tarragon leaves

½ cup extra-virgin olive oil

Salt and freshly ground black pepper

summer chopped *salad*

SERVES 4 TO 6 AS A LIGHT ENTRÉE

This colorful, refreshing salad makes use of summer produce at its peak, and the variety of ingredients, the sweet and spicy pecans, and the fresh tarragon dressing make this something special. Adjust the proportions to your personal taste. I find the more colors in the salad, the more kids like it.

You can find Cajun spice mixture in the spice aisle of your favorite grocery store. Any variety works here. If you don't love tarragon, substitute parsley, cilantro, or dill. —CHEF CRIS

1. **Make the salad:** Spray a large skillet with cooking spray. Heat the pan over medium-high heat and add the corn kernels. Cook, stirring constantly, for about 5 minutes, until the corn is brown in spots. Season with salt and pepper and set aside.

2. Bring a medium saucepan of salted water to a boil. Add the green beans and cook for 1 to 3 minutes; be sure that you don't overcook them—they should still be a little bit crisp. Remove the beans with a slotted spoon and place in a bowl of ice water. Drain, pat dry, and slice into 1-inch pieces. Set aside.

3. **Make the pecans:** Preheat the oven to 250 degrees F. Line a rimmed baking sheet with foil and spray the foil with cooking spray. In a small bowl, toss together the pecans, honey, sugar, melted butter, and Cajun spice mixture. Place on the prepared baking sheet. Bake for 30 minutes, tossing the nuts every 10 minutes, until fragrant and caramelized. Set aside to cool.

4. **Make the dressing:** In a small bowl, combine the vinegar, lemon juice, shallot, and tarragon. Slowly whisk in the olive oil. Season to taste.

5. In a large mixing bowl, place the salad greens, cucumber, radishes, tomatoes, bell pepper, green beans, corn, scallions, and spiced pecans. Pour the dressing over and toss lightly. Serve immediately.

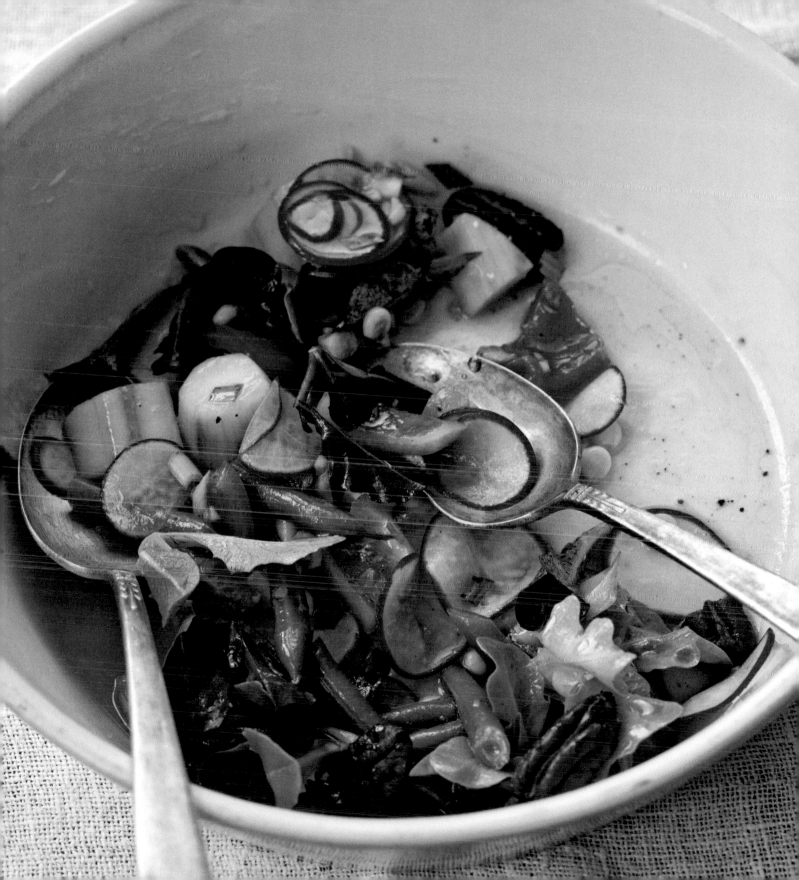

corn soup
with summer vegetables

SERVES 4 TO 6

This versatile soup is the essence of summer. Dairy free and nearly fat free, it showcases the pure, sweet taste of summer corn and can be served hot or at room temperature. A garnish of summer vegetables, grilled and cut into bite-size pieces, makes this soup your own unique creation. Try zucchini or summer squash, tomatoes, eggplant, peppers, or mushrooms, alone or in combination.

If you leave out the corn kernels and don't thin the soup with the corn stock, this becomes a luxurious sauce for seafood like halibut, tilapia, or shrimp. —CHEF SAM

---

4 to 6 ears of fresh corn, shucked and silk removed
2 sprigs fresh thyme
Juice of ½ lemon (about 1 tablespoon)
Salt
Olive oil
Grilled vegetables of your choice: zucchini, summer squash, tomatoes, eggplant, peppers, mushrooms

1. Cut the corn off the cobs and set aside.

2. Place the cobs in a large pot and just barely cover with water. Bring to a boil; then lower the heat and simmer for 45 minutes to 1 hour, until the stock has a rich corn flavor. Strain the stock and set aside.

3. Reserve ¾ cup of the corn kernels and place the remaining corn in a blender. Blend, starting on low speed and increasing the speed as the corn purees. You can add a little of the corn stock to get the corn started. Blend on high for 45 seconds to a minute.

4. Pour the pureed corn into a medium saucepan through a fine-mesh strainer to remove the bits of skin. Add the thyme and cook over medium heat, stirring frequently. You do not want the soup to boil. As the soup heats, the natural starch will begin to thicken the soup. Once the soup has thickened, add the lemon juice and the reserved corn stock little by little until the soup reaches the desired thickness. You should have 4 to 6 cups of soup. Add salt to taste.

5. Heat a small frying pan over medium heat; add enough olive oil to coat the bottom of the pan. When the oil begins to smoke, add the reserved corn kernels and do not stir until the corn has a nice brown color. Stir the corn and then remove it from the heat. Add the seared corn and any other grilled vegetable of your choice on top of the soup and serve.

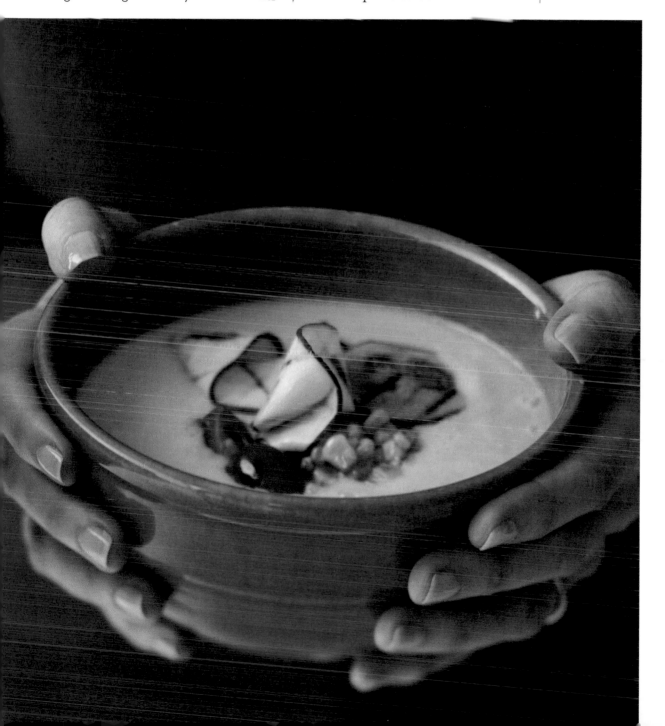

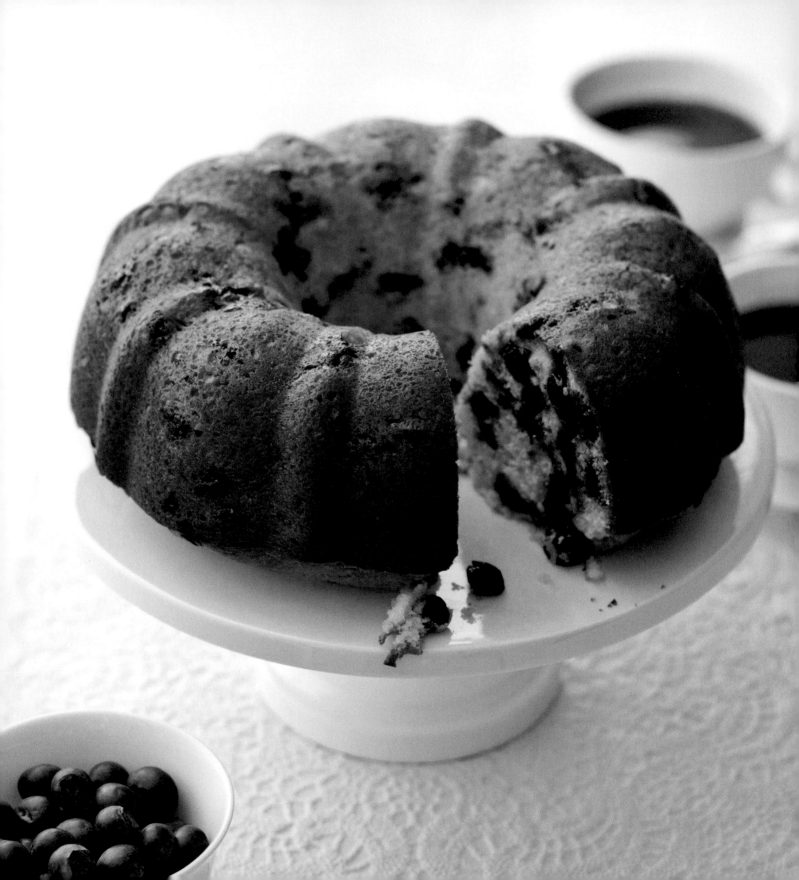

buttermilk *blueberry* bundt cake

SERVES 10 TO 12

We have a competition with the birds on the South Lawn to see who will get to the blueberries first; they are worthy adversaries. In the garden's second year, we built a frame covered in a light mesh over the blueberry bushes to allow water and sunlight to get in but keep the birds out. They still found a way into the little fortress and were able to snatch berries by the beakful.

The blueberries make purple spots throughout the cake and the acidity of the buttermilk contributes to the fine texture of the crumb. If the birds eat all of your blueberries too, you can make this cake with other summer fruits like raspberries, blackberries, or peaches. —CHEF BILL

1. Preheat the oven to 350 degrees F. Grease or spray with cooking spray a 5-quart Bundt pan.

2. Sift the flour, baking powder, salt, and baking soda into a medium bowl.

3. In the bowl of a standing mixer fitted with the paddle attachment, beat the butter and sugar until fluffy and soft.

4. Add the eggs, one at a time, beating well after each addition. Add the vanilla and beat to combine. With the mixer set on low speed, add the flour mixture and buttermilk alternately to the butter mixture. Scrape down the sides between additions.

5. Remove the bowl from the mixer and gently fold in the berries. Scrape the batter into the prepared Bundt pan.

6. Bake for 55 minutes, or until a toothpick inserted near the center of the cake comes out clean. Cool the cake in the pan for at least 20 minutes and then turn out onto a rack to cool completely.

1 cup (2 sticks) unsalted butter, at room temperature, plus additional for greasing the pan
2⅔ cups all-purpose flour
1 tablespoon baking powder
½ teaspoon salt
¼ teaspoon baking soda
1¾ cups sugar
4 large eggs, at room temperature
2 teaspoons pure vanilla extract
½ cup buttermilk
2 pints blueberries, washed and dried

FALL GARDEN HIGHLIGHTS
Tips from Executive Chef Cris Comerford

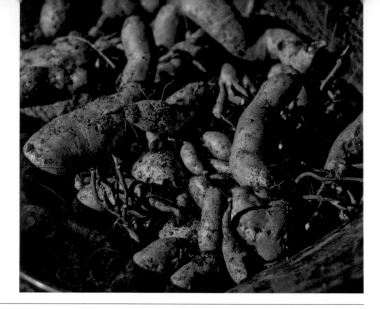

Sweet Potatoes: Many Americans know sweet potatoes as yams, but yams are actually an entirely different plant. Choose potatoes that are firm and do not have cracks, bruises, or spots. Store the potatoes in a cool, dry, dark place, away from heat sources; refrigeration harms their taste. Sweet potatoes that you grow yourself need to be cured for ten days to three weeks (in cold weather) in a warm environment with high humidity. After that, store them in a dark location at about 55 to 60 degrees.

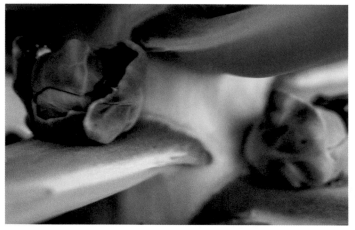

Brussels Sprouts: Brussels sprouts grow on tall leafy stalks, and up close they look like baby cabbages. Recipes and cooking techniques for the sprouts have greatly improved, so they are no longer the bitter, mushy, overcooked vegetable of childhood memories. Brussels sprouts are a cool-weather ripening crop, and the first frost can make them taste sweeter. Look for sprouts that are small, compact, and light green, without any yellowing leaves. Remove any damaged or irregular leaves and store unwashed in plastic bags in the vegetable bin.

Carrots: When selecting fresh carrots, choose ones that are firm, smooth, and relatively straight and bright in color. Limp, rubbery, or cracked carrots are past their prime. If carrots don't have their green tops, make sure that the stem is not dark in color, as this is a sign of age. Thicker carrots are generally sweeter because they have a larger core. Store carrots in the coldest part of the refrigerator, and keep them dry and in a bag. Keep them away from apples, pears, and potatoes, which can cause them to become bitter. In the right conditions, carrots can stay fresh for up to two weeks.

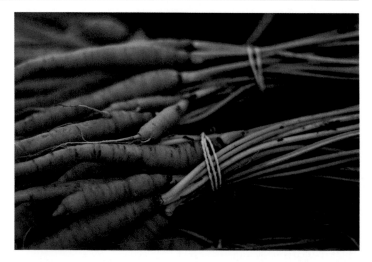

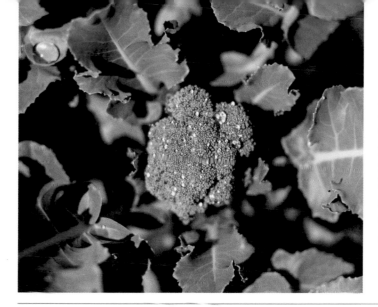

Broccoli: When selecting broccoli, choose floret clusters that are compact and not bruised, with no yellowing. Yellow flowers are a sign that the plant was not harvested soon enough. The stalk and stems should be firm, and there should not be any overly damp or slimy spots on any part of the vegetable. Store broccoli unwashed in a plastic bag in the coldest part of the refrigerator, where it will keep for up to a week.

Cauliflower: When selecting cauliflower, look for a clean, creamy white cap with the bud clusters close together. Brown spots or a dull color are indications of age. Cauliflower should be stored unwashed in a plastic bag in the coldest part of the refrigerator, where it will keep for up to a week. It is best to store it with the head up to keep excess moisture out. Cut cauliflower florets should be eaten within two days. To prepare, remove the outer leaves first and then slice the florets at the base where they meet the stalks. While many traditional cooking methods call for boiling or steaming cauliflower, sautéing preserves more of its flavor and makes it less mushy.

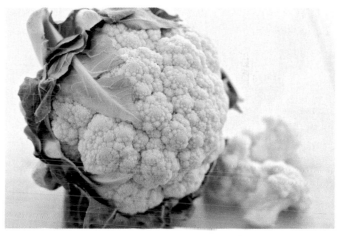

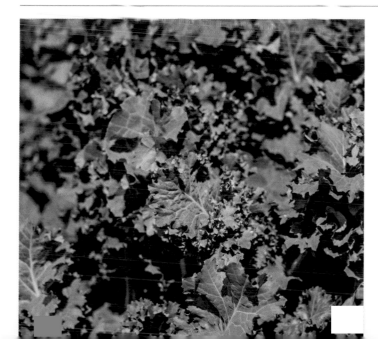

Kale: Kale is easy to grow and thrives in cooler climates; a light frost can produce sweeter leaves. There are several varieties, including curly kale, which has the strongest taste with a peppery flavor; smooth kale, which is sweeter and has a more tender texture; and dinosaur, or Tuscan, kale, which has blue-green leaves. Choose bunches with firm, deeply colored leaves and sturdy stems. Avoid any leaves with browning, yellowing, or small holes. At a store or market, kale needs to be kept in a cool environment; wilted kale has an overly strong taste. Refrigerate unwashed kale in a plastic bag, removing as much of the air as possible. Consume within five days. Longer storage makes its flavor more bitter.

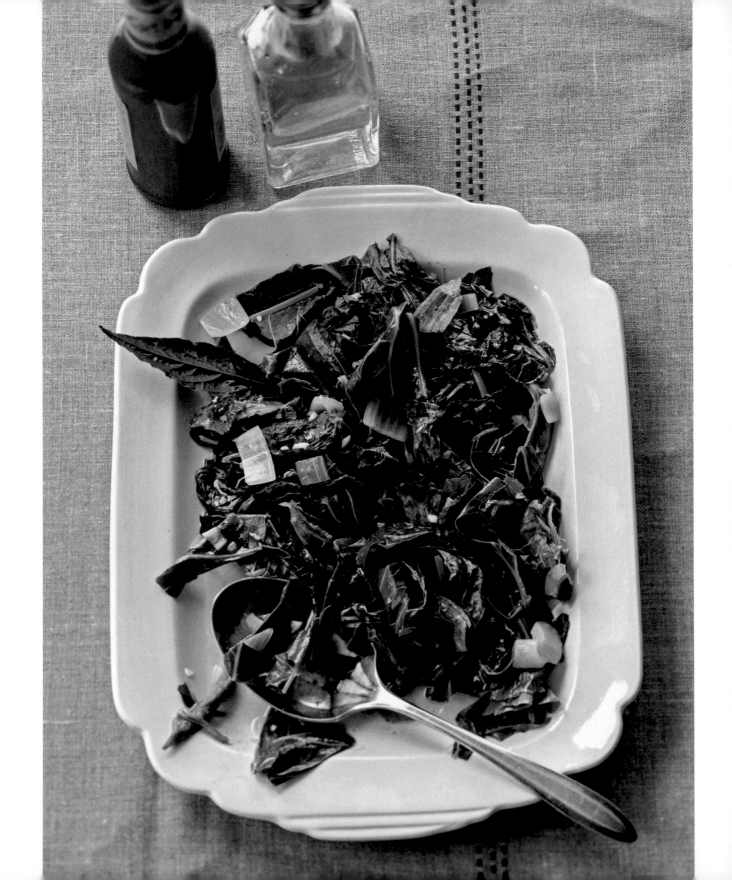

collard *greens*

SERVES 8 TO 10

This not-quite-traditional Southern recipe is a family favorite that has been served at Thanksgiving, as well as at some special private dinners in the White House. Hot sauce is the classic accompaniment and the tang of apple cider vinegar complements the rich, smoky flavor of the greens.

While older recipes call for ham hocks or fatback to be cooked with the greens, my version uses a smoked turkey leg, which adds so much flavor and much less fat to the finished dish. —CHEF CRIS

1. In a large pot, place the smoked turkey leg, bay leaf, quartered onion, and water. Bring to a boil and simmer for about an hour, uncovered. Strain the stock into a large container and set the leg aside to cool. Discard the onion and bay leaf.

2. In a large pot over medium-high heat, drizzle in the olive oil. Add the chopped onion and garlic and cook until translucent, 5 to 7 minutes. Add the collard greens and strained stock and bring to a boil. Lower the heat and cook for about 40 minutes, uncovered, stirring occasionally.

3. Remove the meat from the turkey leg and add it to the pot during the last 5 minutes of cooking. Season with salt and pepper.

4. Serve with your favorite hot sauce and a splash of apple cider vinegar.

1 smoked turkey leg
1 bay leaf
1 onion, quartered
3 quarts water
1 tablespoon extra-virgin olive oil
1 medium onion, finely chopped
6 cloves garlic, minced
2 bunches collard greens (about 2 pounds), well washed, large ribs removed, torn into bite-size pieces
Salt and freshly ground black pepper
Hot sauce, for serving
Apple cider vinegar, for serving

linguine with mushroom bacon sauce

SERVES 6 TO 8

In 2011, in the shade of the trees behind the vegetable garden, we grew our own shiitake mushrooms; you should be able to find them at your local supermarket. The mushrooms have a meaty texture and a depth of flavor that's very satisfying. If you can't find shiitakes, substitute whatever variety is available. The dish will taste a little different but no less delicious.

—CHEF CRIS

1 tablespoon olive oil
1 tablespoon unsalted butter
4 slices bacon, cut into small pieces
6 cloves garlic, minced
1 medium onion, chopped
1½ pounds shiitake mushrooms, stems removed, sliced ¼ inch thick
1 cup half-and-half
½ cup low-sodium chicken stock
1 14.5-ounce box whole-wheat linguine
Zest and juice of 1 lemon
¼ cup chopped fresh flat-leaf parsley
¼ cup grated Parmesan cheese
Salt and freshly ground black pepper

1. In a large saucepan over medium heat, drizzle in the olive oil and add the butter. Add the bacon and cook for about 2 minutes. Add the garlic and onion and cook until translucent, 5 to 7 minutes. Add the mushrooms and cook for about 5 minutes, until fragrant, stirring occasionally.

2. Add the half-and-half and chicken stock and let simmer for about 10 minutes.

3. While the sauce is cooking, bring a large pot of salted water to a boil. Cook the pasta for about 8 minutes, until al dente.

4. Drain the pasta and add it to the saucepan. Add the lemon zest and juice, parsley, and Parmesan. Toss the pasta with the sauce until thoroughly coated. Season with salt and pepper. Serve immediately on a warmed platter.

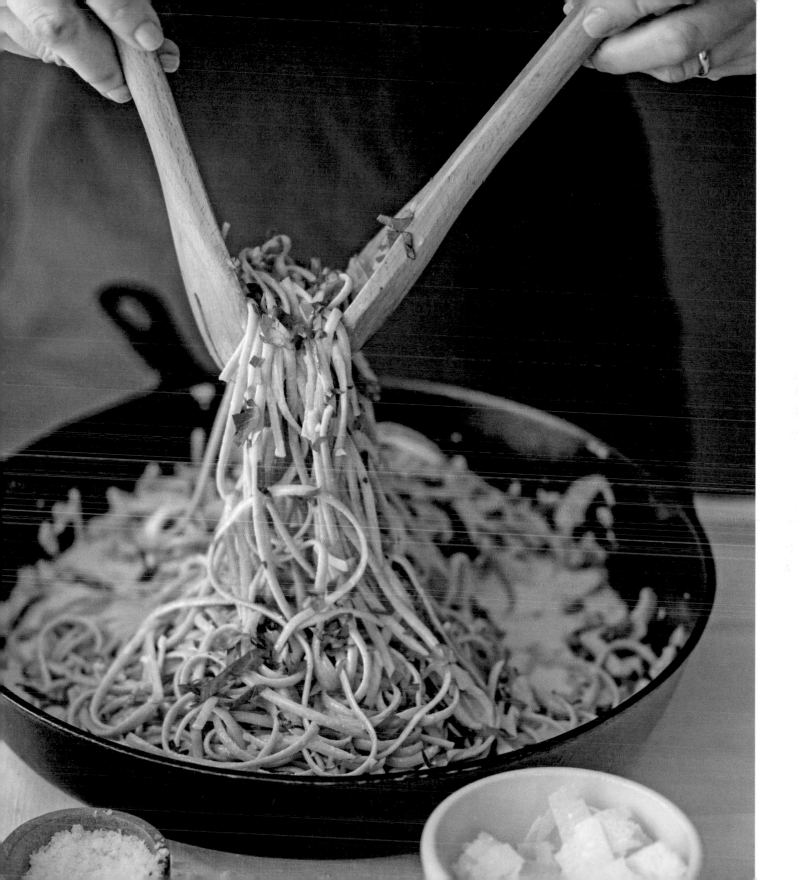

sweet potatoes two ways

SERVES 4 TO 6

No vegetable says fall to me more than sweet potatoes. We've had great luck growing them in the Kitchen Garden, which is a good thing because we're all sweet potato fans here at the White House.

Choose either preparation, whipped or roasted—they're both delicious. If you're cooking for a crowd, just double the quantities.

For the roasted potatoes, I use fresh red chili from the Thomas Jefferson section of our garden; any fresh red chili will do. If you're using chili flakes, add them at the end of the cooking process so they don't burn. A chili's heat is in the seeds; removing them before cooking removes the fire but not the flavor. Both of these dishes taste good and are good for you. —CHEF SAM

ROASTED SWEET POTATOES WITH APPLES AND CHILES

2 sweet potatoes, peeled and cut into bite-size pieces
Olive oil
Salt and freshly ground black pepper
½ Granny Smith or other firm apple, such as Honeycrisp, peeled, cored, and chopped small
1½ teaspoons lemon juice
1 tablespoon unsalted butter (optional)
1 small fresh red chili, stemmed, seeded, and chopped
A pinch of ground cinnamon
½ teaspoon dried chili flakes

1. Preheat the oven to 350 degrees F.

2. Place the sweet potatoes in a bowl and toss with 2 to 3 tablespoons of olive oil; season with salt and pepper. Put the sweet potatoes in one layer on a rimmed baking sheet and cover with foil. Bake until soft, approximately 25 minutes.

3. Drizzle enough olive oil to lightly coat the bottom of a large nonstick frying pan. Place over medium heat. Once the pan is warm, add the sweet potatoes. Be careful not to have the pan too hot; potatoes can easily burn.

4. Gently turn the potatoes with a rubber spatula, until they begin to brown. Add the apple, lemon juice, butter (if using), fresh chili (if using), and cinnamon. Cook until the potatoes are golden brown, continuing to turn the potatoes. Sprinkle with dried chili flakes (if using). Serve immediately.

1. Preheat the oven to 400 degrees F. Place the sweet potatoes in a roasting pan lined with foil and cover with additional foil. Roast for approximately 45 to 60 minutes. The potatoes should be soft all the way through. Remove the potatoes and set aside until they're cool enough to handle.

2. Scoop the potato flesh from the skin into a blender or food processor. Add the butter, orange juice, cinnamon, salt, and nutmeg or allspice (if using). Start to blend on low and slowly increase the speed. If you're using a food processor, pulse 2 or 3 times, then process. You may add a little water or a touch more orange juice to help the potatoes along. Blend or process until smooth and serve.

2 medium sweet potatoes
1½ tablespoons unsalted butter, at room temperature
2 tablespoons orange juice
¼ teaspoon ground cinnamon
Salt to taste
A pinch of nutmeg or allspice (optional)

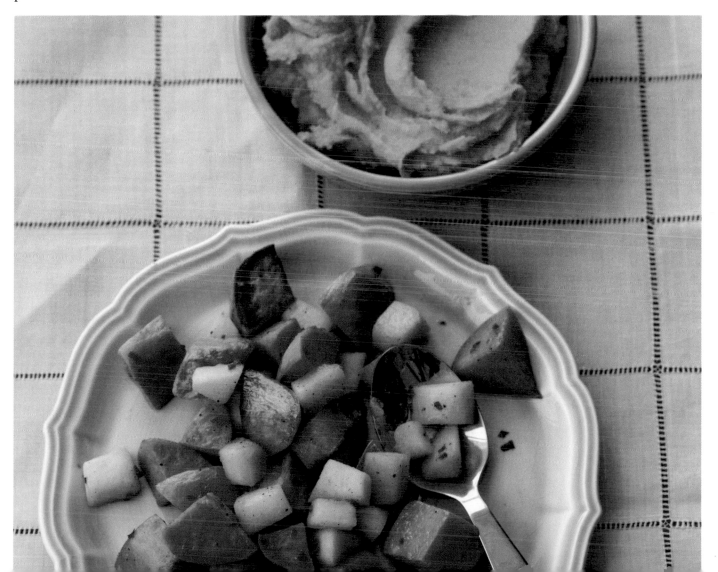

sweet potato quick bread

MAKES TWO 8 x 4-INCH LOAVES

The garden harvest that takes place at the end of summer is one of our favorite events at the White House. Elementary school kids from the Washington, D.C., area who have been our planting partners in the spring return in September to literally reap what they have sown. It is really cool to see the looks on their faces when they realize that the tiny seed they put in the ground now is a plant that is hundreds of times the size of that seed. The grown-ups are pretty impressed too. Mrs. Obama loves to dig up the sweet potatoes with the children; it's a White House treasure hunt!

Try a slice of this not-too-sweet loaf toasted with a smear of cream cheese for breakfast. —CHEF BILL

2 medium sweet potatoes (about 2 pounds)
3 large eggs, at room temperature
¾ cup honey
½ cup canola or other neutral-flavored vegetable oil
½ cup plain Greek yogurt
2½ cups all-purpose flour
1 cup whole-wheat flour
2 teaspoons baking powder
1½ teaspoons salt
2 teaspoons grated fresh ginger
2 tablespoons minced crystallized ginger
2 teaspoons ground ginger

1. Peel the sweet potatoes and cut into large chunks. Place in a medium pot and cover with cold water. Bring to a boil and cook until the potatoes are tender, about 25 to 30 minutes. Drain and puree in a blender or food processor. You should have 2 cups. Set aside to cool.

2. Preheat the oven to 350 degrees F. Grease two 8 ×x 4-inch loaf pans. Cut two strips of parchment paper to the width of the length of each pan; they should be long enough to hang over the edges of the pans. Line the pans with the parchment paper.

3. In a large bowl, mix together the pureed sweet potato, eggs, honey, oil, and yogurt until well blended.

4. In a medium bowl, sift together the all-purpose flour, whole-wheat flour, baking powder, and salt.

5. Add the flour mixture to the sweet potato mixture and combine. Add the gingers and mix until just combined.

6. Spoon the batter into the prepared loaf pans and bake for 1 hour and 15 minutes, or until a toothpick inserted in the center of the loaf comes out clean. Start testing the loaves at 60 minutes.

7. Allow the loaves to cool in the pans for at least 20 minutes before turning out onto a rack to cool completely.

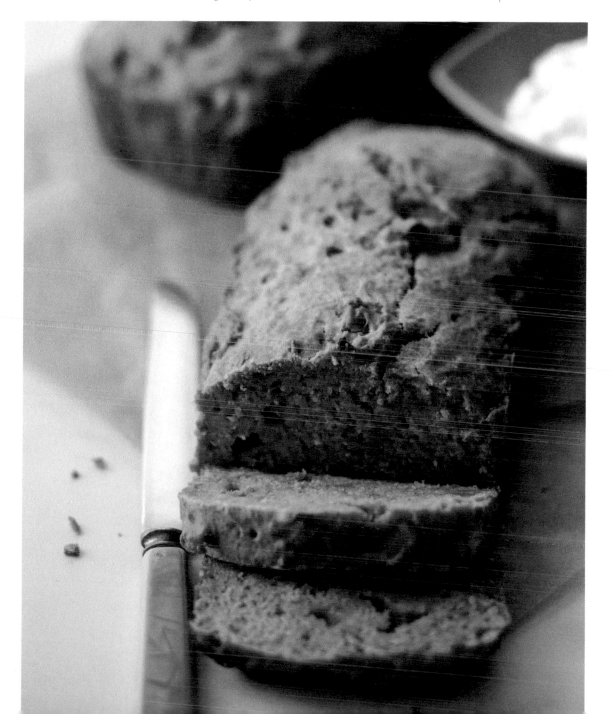

WINTER GARDEN HIGHLIGHTS
Tips from Executive Chef Cris Comerford

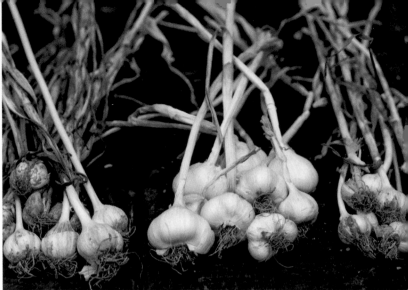

Garlic: In mild climates, garlic can be grown throughout the year, usually by planting individual cloves in the ground. The White House Kitchen Garden grows at least one bed of garlic during the winter. Garlic can be stored at room temperature and keeps longer if the tops remain attached.

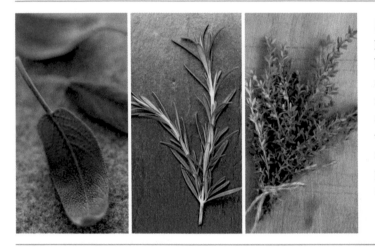

Sage, Rosemary, and Thyme: All three herbs—sage, rosemary, and thyme—are available dried, but the fresh versions have rich flavors and require smaller amounts. Thyme mixes well with eggs, stewed meats, potatoes, beans, fish, and soups. Fresh sage is a classic addition to poultry recipes, and it also works well with eggs and tomato dishes. Rosemary is a favorite seasoning for lamb and chicken dishes, as well as for potatoes, eggs, and tomatoes. Added to olive oil, it can also make a nice dipping sauce for bread.

Beets: Small or medium-size beets are the sweetest and have the best flavor. Beets should be smooth-skinned, with deep colors, and after they are cooked, the skin will peel off easily. Raw beets can be used in salads, if shredded or very thinly sliced. Cut all but two inches of the stems away from the root to prevent moisture loss in the root, and store unwashed in a plastic bag, squeezing out as much air as possible before sealing. Beets may keep for several weeks.

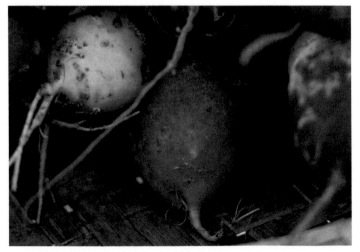

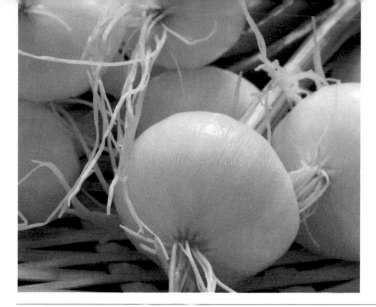

Onions: There are several varieties of onions. Those with dry outer skins are called storage onions and come in red, white, or yellow. They have stronger flavors. Sweet onions, such as Vidalia and Walla Walla, are grown in the spring and summer months. For storage onions, you want dry, crisp skins and no soft spots. Store at room temperature in a well-ventilated space away from heat and light for up to one month.

Collards: Collard greens are quick-growing, taking as little as sixty days from planting to harvest. They are particularly popular in Southern-style cooking, where they are part of a traditional New Year's Day dish, along with black-eyed peas and pork. Collards can also be grown in parts of the North because they can tolerate cooler weather and frost. To achieve the best taste, collards need to be cooked for longer periods than many other greens. They are a good source of vitamins and minerals and can be stored for four or five days in a sealed plastic bag in a refrigerator crisper.

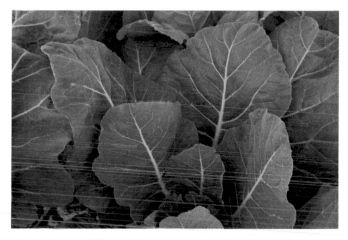

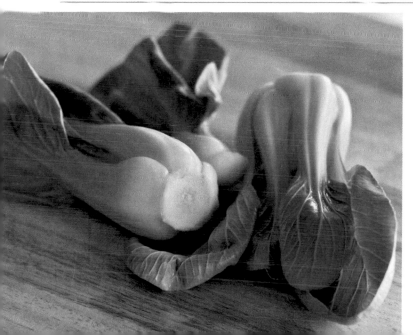

Bok Choy: Bok choy is an Asian cabbage that is rich in vitamins and calcium. Bok choy is used in many Chinese recipes, as well as in Philippine, Thai, and Korean cooking. Smaller plants are more tender and take less time to cook. Bok choy is a cool-weather vegetable and can be stored in the refrigerator. Avoid washing until ready to use.

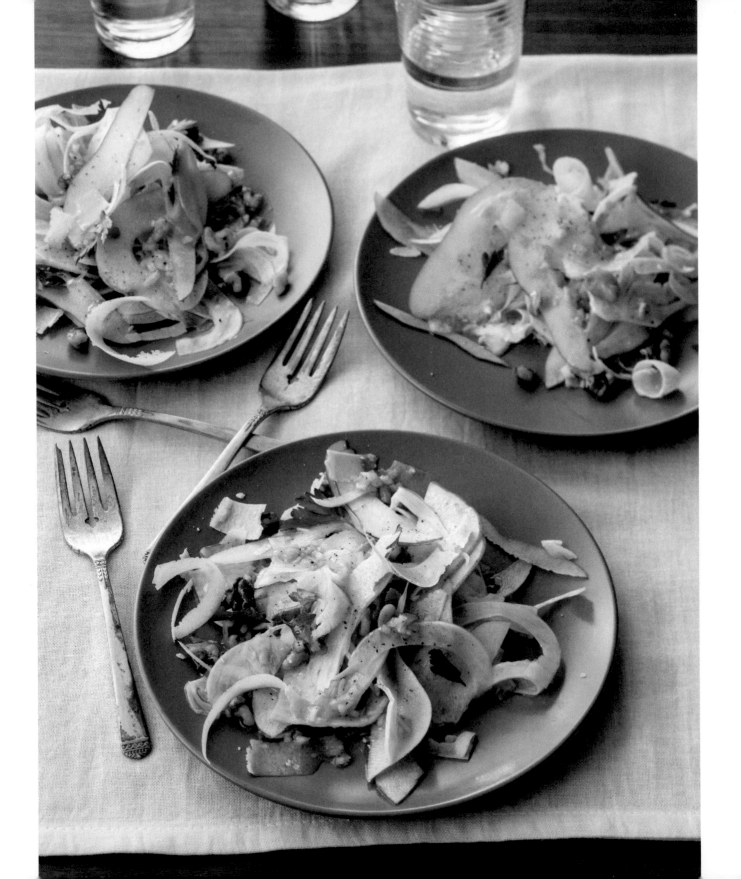

winter *salad*

SERVES 4

The combination of sweet pears, crunchy walnuts, and crunchy fennel makes this salad a winter favorite. Fennel has a similar texture to celery and a sweet licorice-like flavor and is delicious raw in a salad or cooked. You can use any pear you like; Bosc, Anjou, Comice, and Bartlett all will work well. We serve this as a starter at White House lunches and larger receptions because it doesn't wilt or lose its texture while waiting to be eaten. —CHEF CRIS

1. Cut the fennel bulb in half, slice it crosswise into the thinnest possible slices, and set aside.

2. Halve, stem, and core the pear. Slice it to the same thickness as the fennel and then cut the slices into ¼-inch strips. Place in a medium glass or stainless steel mixing bowl and sprinkle with the lemon juice to prevent discoloration. Add the sliced fennel.

3. In a small mixing bowl, add the apple cider vinegar, shallot, and honey. Whisk in the olive oil and season with salt and pepper.

4. Add the vinaigrette and parsley to the fennel and pear mixture. Toss gently. Place on a platter and garnish with the shaved Parmesan cheese and roasted walnuts.

1 fennel bulb, washed and trimmed
1 ripe pear
Juice of ½ lemon (about 1 tablespoon)
1 tablespoon apple cider vinegar
½ shallot, minced
1½ teaspoons honey
4½ teaspoons extra-virgin olive oil
Salt and freshly ground black pepper
1½ teaspoons chopped fresh flat-leaf parsley
2 ounces Parmesan cheese, shaved
½ cup roasted walnuts

cauliflower *mac and cheese*

SERVES 3 OR 4

Using pureed cauliflower gives this variation on the classic mac and cheese a deliciously creamy texture without the extra fat and calories, and the whole-wheat pasta has a nutty flavor. The pasta and cauliflower can be cooked at the same time, and since you're not baking the dish, it's an easy weeknight treat. Serve it as a side; or just add a salad and you've got dinner. If you're feeding a family with big appetites, the recipe is easily doubled. —CHEF CRIS

1. Bring a large pot of salted water to a boil and cook the pasta according to the package directions until al dente. Drain and set aside.

2. Bring a medium pot of salted water to a boil, add the cauliflower, and cook for 5 to 7 minutes, or until soft. Drain. Place the cauliflower in a blender and puree.

3. In a medium pan over medium heat, place the pasta, the cauliflower puree, the cheeses, and the milk. Stir gently to combine and continue stirring until the cheese is melted.

4. Season with salt and pepper. Sprinkle the chopped parsley over the mac and cheese and serve immediately.

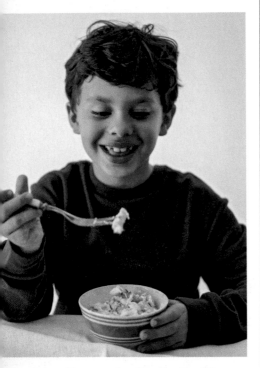

Theo, a student from Brooklyn PS 107 (see page 140).

½ pound whole-wheat penne
¼ head cauliflower, cut into florets
8 ounces sharp Cheddar cheese, shredded
1 ounce Parmesan cheese, grated
½ cup 1% or 2% milk
Salt and freshly ground black pepper
1½ teaspoons chopped fresh flat-leaf parsley

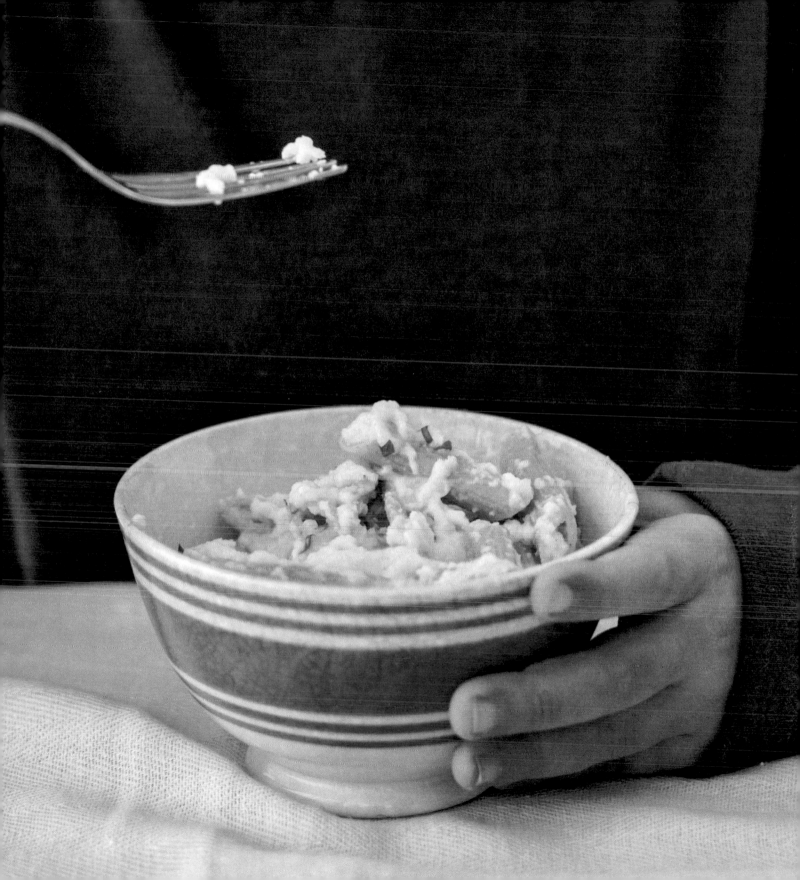

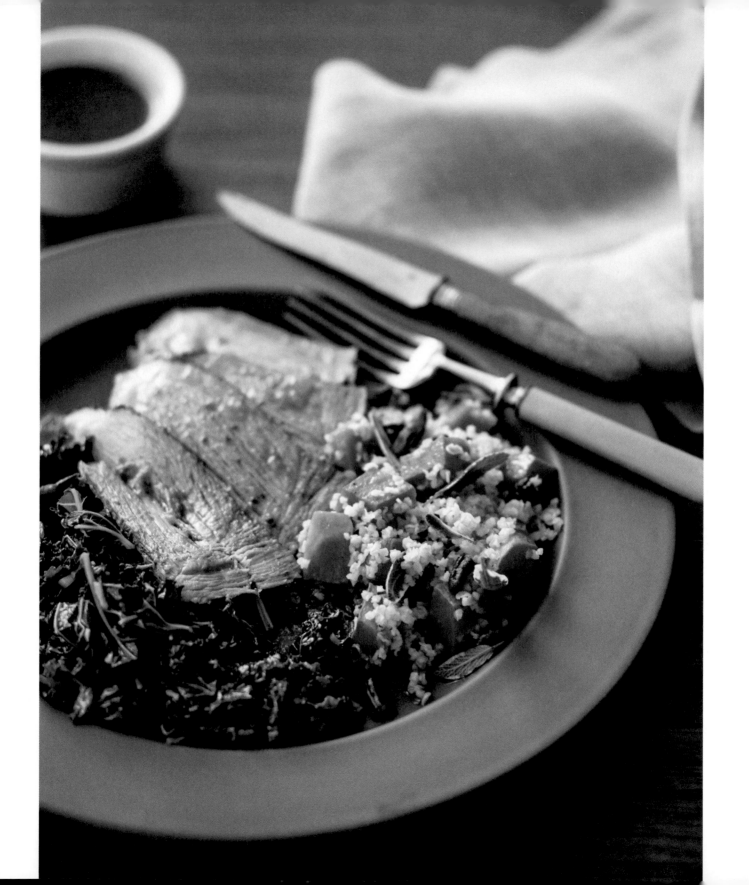

braised *pork shoulder* with butternut squash and greens

SERVES 8 TO 10, WITH LEFTOVER PORK

Here's a complete dinner for a cold Sunday night. The meat cooks largely unattended; you could even make it the day before and reheat it when you're ready to eat.

This is an economical meal that will feed a crowd. If you have leftover pork, shred it, cover it with the remaining liquid, and refrigerate or freeze. It can be the start for any number of delicious bonus dishes: Add it to tomato sauce to serve over pasta; use it to flavor fried rice; combine it with barbecue sauce and pile the meat on a bun; or add it to a pot of cooked beans.

Don't throw away the seeds from the squash. You can prepare them just like pumpkin seeds for a crunchy snack (page 257). —CHEF SAM

1. **Make the pork:** Heat a large pot over high heat. When hot, coat with vegetable oil and sear the pork shoulder on all sides until dark brown. Remove and set aside.

2. Add the carrots to the pot and cook for 2 to 3 minutes; then add the onion, garlic, bay leaves, poblano and ancho chilies, and the chili powder. Cook until there is some color on the vegetables.

3. Place the pork shoulder back in the pot and add the stock and salt. Add water until the shoulder is just covered by the liquid. Bring to a boil and reduce the heat to a simmer. Cover and cook for 2½ to 3 hours; the meat should be fork-tender and easily come off the bone. Set aside.

4. **Make the squash:** About 30 minutes before serving, preheat the oven to 375 degrees F. Line a rimmed baking sheet with foil. In a medium bowl, toss the squash with a little olive oil and a sprinkle of salt and spread in a

RECIPE CONTINUES

FOR THE PORK
Vegetable oil
1 4-pound pork shoulder, excess
   fat removed
2 carrots, peeled and diced
1 onion, diced
5 cloves garlic
3 bay leaves
2 poblano chilies, stemmed,
   seeded, and diced
2 ancho chilies, stemmed,
   seeded, and diced or
   2 tablespoons ancho chili
   powder
1 tablespoon chipotle chili powder
6 cups low-sodium chicken stock
1½ tablespoons salt

FOR THE SQUASH
1 small butternut squash, peeled,
   seeded, and cut into 1-inch
   cubes
¼ cup olive oil, plus more for
   tossing the squash
Salt
1 cup bulgur wheat
2½ cups boiling water
2 to 3 tablespoons chopped sage
½ cup chopped toasted pecans

single layer on the baking sheet. Cover with foil and roast for 20 minutes, or until soft.

FOR THE GREENS
2 tablespoons olive oil
1 clove garlic, chopped
1 bunch kale, collard greens, or Swiss chard, washed, large ribs removed, and cut into bite-size pieces
1 cup braising liquid from pork shoulder
Salt and freshly ground black pepper

5. Meanwhile, place the bulgur wheat in a medium heat-proof bowl. Add the boiling water and let sit for approximately 20 minutes. Add the roasted squash, sage, pecans, and a little olive oil and stir gently to combine.

6. When the pork is cooled, remove the meat and set aside. Strain the stock and discard the vegetables and bay leaves. Let the stock stand for a few minutes, until the fat rises to the top of the container; skim the fat and return the stock to the pot. Reduce the stock over medium heat for 10 to 15 minutes; add salt to taste.

7. **Make the greens:** In a large saucepan over medium-high heat, heat the olive oil. Add the garlic and cook until light brown; do not burn.

8. Add the kale and stir to coat with the oil and garlic. Add the braising liquid and bring to a boil. Lower the heat and simmer for 10 minutes, or until tender. Season with salt and pepper.

9. Slice the meat, discarding any bones. Pour the remaining braising liquid over the meat and serve with the squash and greens.

roasted *pumpkin seeds*

This is more of a technique than a recipe, as the amounts of ingredients will depend on the amount of seeds you have. You can use seeds from winter squashes like butternut or acorn squash just like pumpkin seeds.

Scoop the seeds out of your pumpkin (or squash) and place in a pot. Add enough water to cover the seeds by one inch and add a tablespoon of salt. Bring the water to a boil, and boil the seeds for 15 to 20 minutes. Drain the seeds in a strainer and rinse with cold water. Most of the pumpkin flesh will have dissolved; now's the time to remove the rest. Don't worry if a little clings to the seeds. Blot the seeds to remove excess moisture.

Preheat the oven to 350 degrees F. Line a rimmed baking sheet with foil and spray the foil with cooking spray. Dump the seeds onto the pan; drizzle with a little olive oil and spread the seeds out over the pan. Bake the seeds for 10 to 15 minutes, or until they become crunchy and light brown; start checking after 8 minutes to make sure the seeds don't burn.

You can add any herbs or spices to the seeds after you add the olive oil, but you won't need salt.

white chocolate–cherry–*carrot* cookies

MAKES APPROXIMATELY 24 COOKIES

The White House Kitchen Garden is a bonanza for the main kitchen, but the pastry kitchen mainly uses the rhubarb, sweet potatoes, and carrots. (We do get the lion's share of the fresh honey from the beehive, though.) Because we love all things Hawaiian at the White House, I use macadamia nuts in this cookie; pecans or walnuts can be substituted, as can dried cranberries for the dried cherries. —CHEF BILL

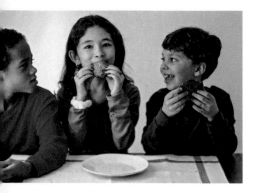

Aidan, Tamaris, and Theo, students at Brooklyn PS 107 (see page 140).

1¾ cups all-purpose flour
1 teaspoon baking powder
½ teaspoon salt
1 cup (2 sticks) unsalted butter, at room temperature
1¼ cups (packed) light brown sugar
1 tablespoon mild honey
2 teaspoons pure vanilla extract
2 large eggs
1 cup dried cherries
¼ cup toasted chopped macadamia nuts (optional)
2 ounces white chocolate, chopped into small pieces, or white chocolate chips
1 cup finely grated carrots

1. Preheat the oven to 350 degrees F. Place the rack in the center of the oven.

2. Sift together the flour with the baking powder and salt. Set aside.

3. In the large bowl of an electric mixer, beat together the butter, brown sugar, honey, and vanilla until smooth. Add the eggs and mix until well combined. Scrape down the bowl.

4. On low speed, add the cherries, nuts, and chocolate. Scrape down the bowl.

5. Stop the mixer and add one-third of the flour mixture. Turn to low speed and combine. Stop the mixer again, add the rest of the flour mixture, and combine on low speed.

6. Add the carrots, and mix on low speed until incorporated. The batter will be stiff.

7. Using a standard ice cream scoop or a heaped tablespoon, drop batter in mounds, 2 inches apart, onto a parchment-covered cookie sheet.

8. Bake for 12 to 14 minutes, remove from the oven, and allow the cookies to cool completely before removing them from the cookie sheet.

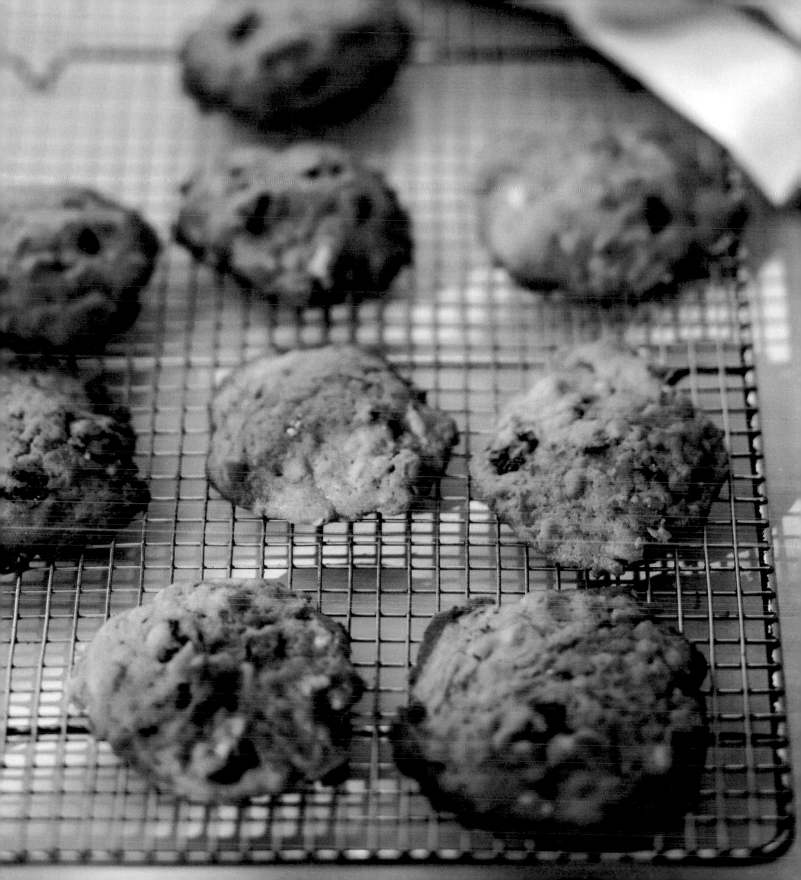

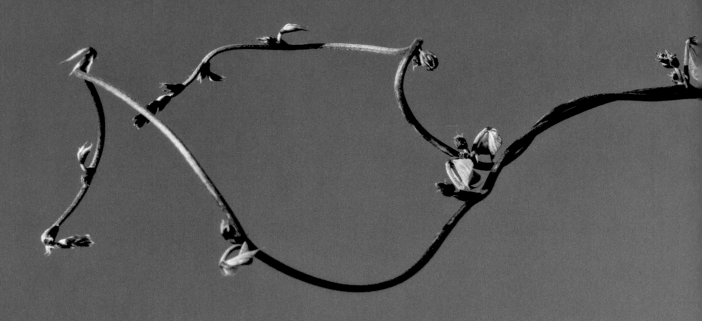

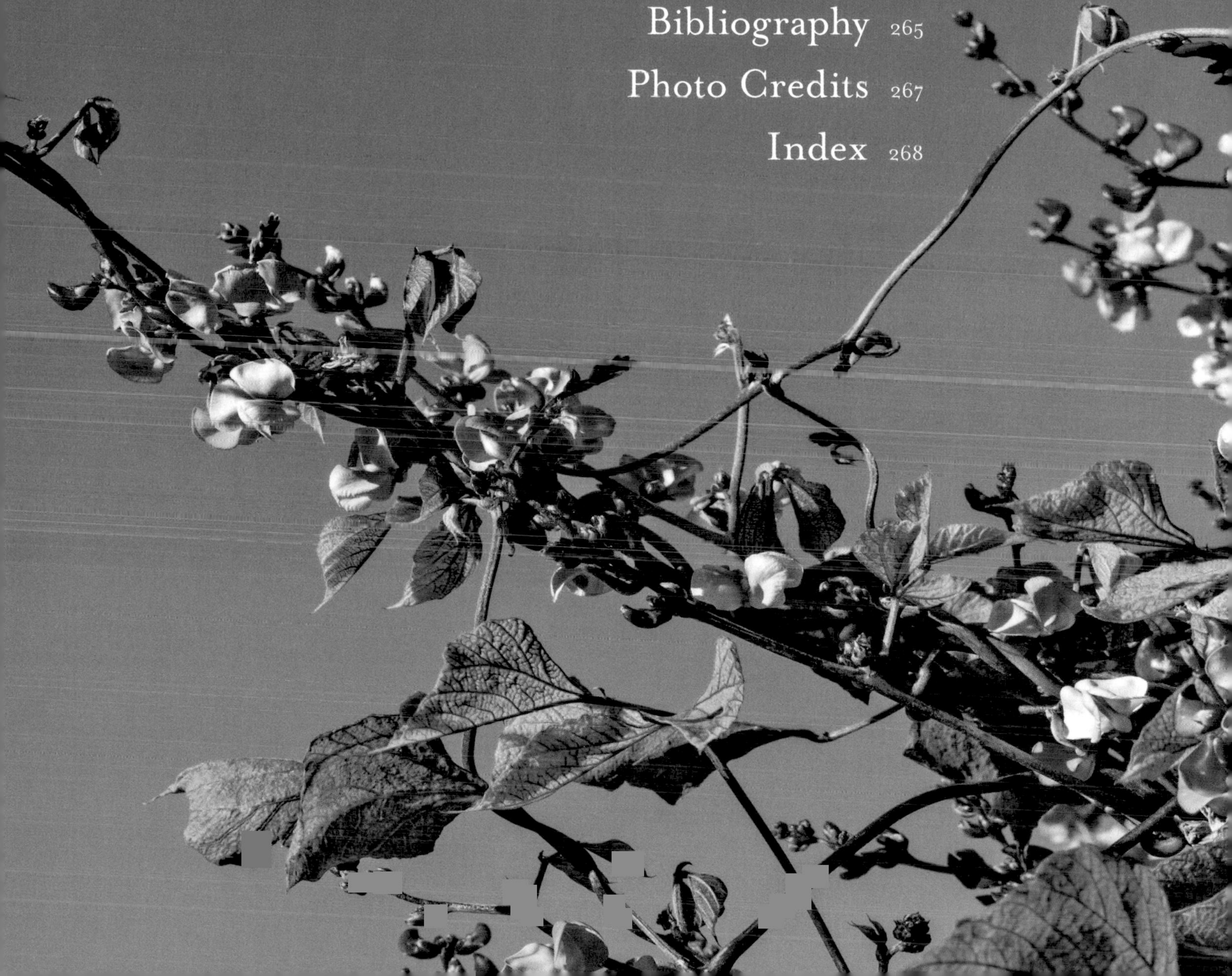

ACKNOWLEDGMENTS

I want to express my deepest gratitude to the following people for their commitment to encouraging healthy living and their work to make this book possible.

To Jim Adams; James Pilkerton; and Jessica Amerson and the many National Park Service staff; and Dale Haney, the White House groundskeeper; who help support the Kitchen Garden and care for the White House grounds. I truly appreciate their dedication to preserving our nation's most beautiful places and their willingness to share their vast knowledge with me and all those who visit our garden.

To Charlie Brandts, our beekeeper in chief. Charlie has worked at the White House for almost three decades, and his passion for beekeeping has been essential to our garden's success.

To the White House chefs, Cris Comerford, Bill Yosses, and Sam Kass. Cris's dedication to providing healthy meals for our guests and helping other moms provide healthy meals for their families truly inspires me. Bill never ceases to amaze me with his imaginative treats and generosity of spirit. And I cannot thank Sam enough for his tireless work to improve the health of children and families all across our country.

To Bill Allman, White House Curator, for sharing the living history of the White House with our family and so many others, and to the White House Historical Association for their devoted efforts to enhance and preserve this national treasure.

To Peter Hatch, Director of Gardens and Grounds at President Jefferson's Monticello home, who taught us so much about a great American President and gardener. A special thanks for carrying on President Jefferson's tradition of sharing seeds from his garden to plant in our White House Kitchen Garden.

To Steve Badt and Miriam's Kitchen for providing quality services and support to those in need in our D.C. community. I am grateful for the opportunities they have given us to volunteer and to donate so much of our garden produce for the healthy, delicious meals they serve.

To Chef Dan Barber, Jim Crawford, and the many others who guided us, for their support and leadership.

To our friends at the U.S. Department of Agriculture, Department of Health and Human Services, Department of the Interior, and the White House Domestic Policy Council, as well as everyone in the Office of the First Lady and throughout the White House whose expertise, enthusiasm, and hard work is helping to lift up families and communities all across America.

To Maya Mavjee, Tina Constable, Sydny Miner, Marysarah Quinn, Lyric Winik, Quentin Bacon, Bob Barnett, and the Crown Publishing Group team for their valuable experience and guidance and for helping me share these stories with others.

To the educators and students at Bancroft Elementary School and Harriet Tubman Elementary School for helping us plant and harvest the garden right from the beginning and for filling the garden with joy and wonder.

To all the gardeners, schools, businesses, and organizations featured in this book for sharing their stories and knowledge and for helping to build and continue this movement.

To the many volunteers who have provided everything from cooking lessons to construction advice and who have stepped onto the South Lawn, gotten their hands dirty, and lovingly tended this garden as if it were their own.

To all the parents and children who are working every day to make changes at home and in their communities.

To the businesses and organizations that have answered our call to help raise a healthier generation of young people.

And finally, to my husband and daughters, and our friends and family, whose love and support lifts and sustains me every step of the way. And, of course, to our dog, Bo, who faithfully watches over the garden and kindly refrains from digging up the vegetables.

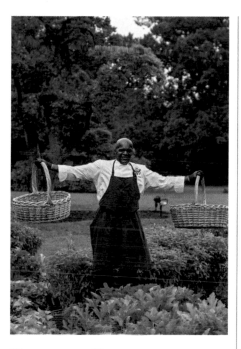

HEALTH AND NUTRITION

Let's Move!: A comprehensive website with information on physical activity and healthy eating and resources for parents, caregivers, educators, community leaders, and others interested in helping our children lead healthier lives. www.letsmove.gov

Chefs Move! to Schools: Includes stories from chefs who participate and information about how chefs can sign up to partner with schools and how schools can sign up to locate a willing volunteer chef. www.chefsmovetoschools.org

President's Council on Fitness Sports & Nutrition: Provides ideas and incentives for maintaining a healthy lifestyle with physical activity and good nutrition. It also offers the President's Challenge and fitness awards, including the Presidential Active Lifestyle Award and the Presidential Champions Challenge. www.fitness.gov

HealthierUS School Challenge: A voluntary program for schools participating in the National School Lunch Program. To be eligible, schools must improve the quality of the food they serve, provide students with nutrition education, and offer physical education and opportunities for physical activity. Monetary incentive awards are available for each HUSSC award level: Bronze, Silver, Gold, and the Gold Award of Distinction. Applications are available at the link below and may be submitted by U.S. mail or online. If two or more schools from one school district are applying, a simplified district application process is available. www.teamnutrition.usda .gov/HealthierUS/index.html

MyPlate/MiPlato: Offers tips on how to achieve a healthy balance of foods on your plate. For more information on healthy food choices, in English or in Spanish, visit www.choosemy plate.gov/ and www.choosemyplate .gov/en-espanol.html

Farm to School: A USDA initiative that connects K–12 schools with regional or local farms to help them serve healthy meals using locally produced foods. For information on applications, guidelines, and eligibility, go to www.fns.usda.gov/cnd/f2s/

Know Your Farmer, Know Your Food: The U.S. Department of Agriculture launched the Know Your Farmer, Know Your Food initiative in 2009. This initiative brings together staff from across the USDA to coordinate, share resources, and publicize USDA efforts related to local and regional food systems. www.usda.gov/wps/portal/ usda/usdahome?navid-HOME&navtype=MA

There are many kinds of nutrition and nutrition supplement programs at the USDA. They provide ways for seniors to access farmers' markets and schools to access fresh fruits and vegetables and better breakfasts. Here are links to some of the most popular programs:

Farmers' Market Nutrition Program: www.fns.usda.gov/fmnp

Senior Farmers' Market Nutrition Program: www.fns.usda.gof/sfmnp

USDA Fresh Fruit and Vegetable Program for Schools: www.fns.usda.gov/ffvp

USDA School Breakfast Program: www.fns.usda.gov/breakfast

Team Nutrition (aimed at children, with special information for caregivers): www.fns.usda.gov/tn

USDA Summer Food Service Program: www.fns.usda.gov/sfsp

GARDENING

U.S. Department of Agriculture's People's Garden Initiative: What began as an effort to challenge USDA employees to create gardens at the Department's facilities has since grown into a collaborative effort of more than seven hundred local and national organizations all working together to establish community and school gardens across the country. Learn how to start a People's Garden and find practical gardening advice, resources, grant information, recipes, and more on the USDA website at www.usda.gov/peoplesgarden.

USDA Master Gardener Program: Get advice from a USDA master gardener, or even get trained as a master gardener yourself through the USDA. Learn about community gardening, environmental gardening, and youth gardening, among other topics. Master gardeners volunteer their time to help Americans plant, grow, and harvest fresh produce from their gardens. Find resources created by the Extension Master Gardener community at www.extension.org/mastergardener

Find an Extension Master Gardener program in every state, Washington, D.C., and Canada at www.extension.org/9925.

The Junior Master Gardener (JMG) Program is an international youth gardening program operated nationwide through the Cooperative Extension network. JMG is "Growing Good Kids" by igniting a passion for learning, success, and service. Be a part of JMG at www.jmgkids.us

USDA Cooperative Extension Program: Connects you to USDA experts at state land-grant universities and local and regional offices that can provide useful, practical information on gardening and nutrition. The Cooperative Extension System is a nationwide, noncredit educational network. Each U.S. state and territory has a state office at its land-grant university and a network of local or regional offices. The USDA's National Institute of Food and Agriculture (NIFA) is the federal partner in the Cooperative Extension System. For general information on the USDA Cooperative Extension Program, and to locate your nearest Cooperative Extension office, visit www.nifa.usda.gov/Extension/index.html

For more information on starting a community garden, see this "how-to" guide from the University of California's Cooperative Extension program: celosangeles.ucdavis.edu/Common_Ground_Garden_Program/Community_Gardens.html

For guidance about what plants grow best in what climate, check out the USDA Plant Hardiness Zone Map at www.usna.usda.gov/Hardzone/

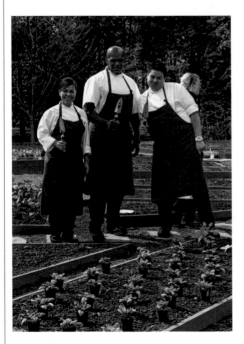

BIBLIOGRAPHY

BOOKS

Betts, Edwin Morris, ed. *Thomas Jefferson's Garden Book, 1766–1824: With Relevant Extracts from His Other Writings*. Philadelphia, PA: American Philosophical Society, 1944.

Bucklin-Sporer, Arden, and Rachel Kathleen Pringle. *How to Grow a School Garden: A Complete Guide for Parents and Teachers*. Portland, OR: Timber Press, 2010.

Graham, Wade. *American Eden: From Monticello to Central Park to Our Backyards: What Our Gardens Tell Us About Who We Are*. New York: HarperCollins, 2011.

Grohsgal, Brett, and Julia Shanks. *The Farmer's Kitchen: The Ultimate Guide to Enjoying Your CSA and Farmers' Market Foods*. Cambridge, MA: CSA Cookbooks, 2011.

Hatch, Peter J. *The Gardens of Thomas Jefferson's Monticello*. Charlottesville, VA: Thomas Jefferson Memorial Foundation, 1992.

Hatch, Peter J. *"A Rich Spot of Earth": Thomas Jefferson's Revolutionary Garden at Monticello*. With a foreword by Alice Waters. New Haven, CT: Yale University Press, 2012.

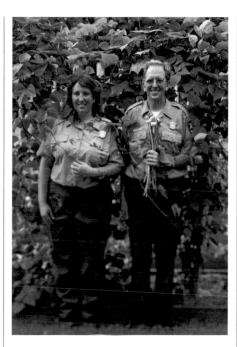

Johnson, Lady Bird, and Carlton B. Lees. *Wildflowers Across America*. Austin, TX: National Wildlife Research Center, New York, NY: Abbeville Press, 1998.

Kirby, Ellen, and Elizabeth Peters, eds. *Community Gardening: Brooklyn Botanic Garden All-Region Guides*. Brooklyn, NY: Brooklyn Botanic Garden, 2009.

Lawson, Laura J. *City Bountiful: A Century of Community Gardening in America*. Berkeley: University of California Press, 2005.

Loewer, Peter. *Jefferson's Garden*. Mechanicsburg, PA: Stackpole Books, 2004.

Seale, William. *The President's House: A History*, 2nd ed., vols. 1 and 2. Baltimore: Johns Hopkins University Press in association with the White House Historical Association, 2008.

Seale, William. *The White House Garden*. Washington, DC: The White House Historical Association, 1996.

Smith, Edward C. *The Vegetable Gardener's Bible*, 2nd ed. North Adams, MA: Storey, 2009.

Smith, Jeremy N. *Growing a City Garden: How Farmers, First Graders, Counselors, Troubled Teens, Foodies, A Homeless Shelter Chef, Single Mothers, and More Are Transforming Themselves and Their Neighborhoods Through the Intersection of Local Agriculture and Community—and How You Can, Too*. With a foreword by Bill McKibben. New York: Skyhorse, 2010.

Stell, Elizabeth P. *Secrets to Great Soil: A Grower's Guide to Composting, Mulching, and Creating Healthy, Fertile Soil for Your Garden and Lawn*. North Adams, MA: Storey, 1998.

Thomas, Robert B. *The Old Farmer's Almanac, 2011*. Dublin, NH: Yankee, 2011.

Tucker, David M. *Kitchen Gardening in America: A History*. Ames: Iowa State University Press, 1993.

Wulf, Andrea. *Founding Gardeners: The Revolutionary Generation, Nature, and the Shaping of the American Nation.* New York: Alfred A. Knopf, 2011.

WEBSITES

Let's Move!: www.letsmove.gov

Obama Foodorama: The Blog of Record About White House Food Initiatives, from Policy to Pie: www.obamafoodorama.blogspot.com

USA Today: www.usatoday.com

The Washington Post: www.washington post.com

Renee's Garden: www.reneesgarden .com. See the article by Alice Formiga, "Celebrate the Three Sisters: Corn, Beans, and Squash."

JOURNALS AND CATALOGS

White House Historical Association: www.whha.org

Johnny's Selected Seeds. 2011/2012. Winslow, Maine.

High Mowing Organic Seeds. 2012. Wolcott, Vermont.

D. Landreth Seed Company. 2012. New Freedom, Pennsylvania.

SiteLines: A Journal of Place 6, no. 11 (Spring 2011).

Additional resources and assistance provided by: Lady Bird Johnson Wildflower Center, Library of Congress; Department of Agricultural History, Iowa State University, Ames; Department of History, Michigan Technological University, Houghton;

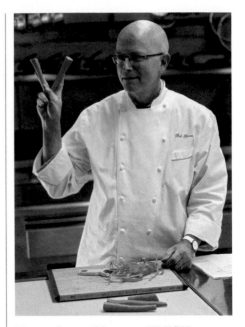

NatureSpace Chicago; FRESH-FARM Markets, Washington, DC; New Morning Farm Farmers' Markets and New Morning Farm, Huston, PA; Lafayette Farmers' Market, Washington, DC; Redbud Organic Farm, Inwood, WV; Smith Meadows Farm, Berryville, VA; Even' Star Organic Farm, Lexington Park, MD; and Nob Hill Orchards, Gerrardstown, WV; North Carolina Cooperative Extension and 4-H; Maya Angelou Institute for the Improvement of Child and Family Education, Winston-Salem State University, Winston-Salem, NC; City of Houston, TX; and the International Rescue Committee, San Diego, CA.

DEDICATION TO THE GARDEN
The entire White House grounds are a national park, and the National Park Service devotes considerable care to them. We are lucky to have Park Service expertise in the garden.

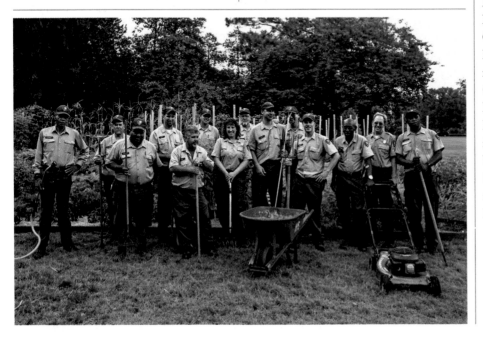

PHOTO CREDITS

Rana Abu-Sbaih: page 139 (bottom left)

Dan Allen: pages 90 (right), 91 (all)

Amoret Tanner Collection / The Art Archive at Art Resource, NY: page 177

AP Photo: pages 29 (right), 183

Official White House Photo by Samantha Appleton: pages 8, 17, 56 (left), 178, 196 (top)

Koji Aoki/AFLO/Getty Images: page 201 (bottom)

Quentin Bacon Photography: pages 1, 2, 4, 5, 6, 22, 24, 27 (present-day White House photo), 34 (all), 35 (all), 37 (all), 38, 39 (all), 40, 41 (bottom left and bottom right), p. 42 (all), 43 (all), 44, 46 (bottom), 47 (all), 49 (all), 50 (top left), 51 (bottom left, bottom right), 52 (all), 53, 60, 61 (all), 62 (all), 64 (left, top right), 65, 66 (all), 67 (all), 68 (all), 69, 72–73, 74 (all), 75 (all), 76 (all), 77 (all), 78–79, 80–81, 82, 84, 85, 86, 87 (all), 98, 99 (all), 100, 102 (top left, bottom left), 103 (all), 104–105 (all), 106 (all), 107 (all), 110–111, 112 (all), 113 (all), 114 (all), 115 (all), 116–117, 118–119, 120, 122 (all), 123, 124 (all), 127 (left), 128–129, 130 (all), 132, 133, 136, 147, 148, 150, 151 (all), 154–155, 156 (all), 157 (all), 158 (all), 159 (all), 160–161, 162, 163, 164, 166, 167, 168, 169 (all), 170, 171 (all), 202, 206–207, 208 (all), 209 (all), 210–211, 214, 215, 216–217, 218 (all), 219 (top, bottom), 221, 223, 224, 227, 228 (all), 229 (all), 230, 233, 235, 236, 238 (all), 239 (top, bottom), 240, 243, 245, 247, 248 (top, bottom), 250, 252, 253, 254, 257, 258, 259, 260–261, 263, 264, 265, 266 (all), 272

Eric Ballhaussen: page 186 (all)

Bettmann/CORBIS: pages 26 (top and bottom), 27 (inset)

Richard Bloom/Getty Images: page 149 (right)

AP Photo/Alex Brandon: page 179 (bottom right)

Rosemary Calvert/Getty Images: page 59

Maren Caruso/Digital Vision/ Getty Images: page 249 (bottom)

AP Photo/Manuel Balce Ceneta: pages 55, 179 (top right)

Manuel Balce Ceneta/AP/Corbis: page 199

Chicago Historical Museum: page 13

Stephen Conroy /the food passionates/Corbis: page 50 (bottom)

Jeffrey Coolidge/Riser/Getty Images: page 248 (middle center)

Shealah Craighead: page 191

Stephen Crowley/The New York Times: page 31

Dr. Beth Day-Hairston: page 95 (right)

Peter Dazeley/ Getty Images: page 180

Earl B. Depue: page 101 (bottom)

Sandra Deshotel: pages 88 (top), 89 (all)

Andrew Dernie/Getty Images: page 62 (bottom)

Mike Devlin: page 135 (right)

AP Photo/Charles Dharapak: pages 20–21, 41 (top left), 181 (all)

Joseph Domin / Chicago Historical Museum: page 12

Harrison Eastwood/Getty Images: page 195 (right)

Mary E. Eaton/National Geographic Society/Corbis: page 50 (top right)

Jonathan Ernst/Reuters/Corbis: page 16

REUTERS/Jonathan Ernst: page 54

Valerie Frick: page 134 (left)

Geography and Maps Division, Library of Congress: page 25

Getty Images: page 62 (bottom)

AP Photo/Haraz N. Ghanbari: page 179 (bottom left)

Seve Ghose: page 197 (bottom)

Courtesy of Growing Power: pages 144, 145 (all)

SELCAN HACAOGLU/AP/Corbis: page 174

Ryan Harvey Photography/Digital Vision/Getty Images: page 248 (middle left)

Kaye Hausen: page 94 (left)

Ben Helphand: page 93 (all)

Historic American Buildings Survey, Prints & Photographs, Library of Congress: page 28

Historical Picture Archive/ CORBIS: page 51 (top)

AP Photo/Nam Y. Huh: page 149 (left)

Huntstock/Getty Images: page 58

Icon Sports Media/Corbis: page 201 (top)

Michele Israel: pages 140 (all), 141 (all)

Photography by Jess Jackson: page 139 (top right, bottom right)

Official White House Photo by Lawrence Jackson: pages 96, 97, 142, 192 (all), 193

Susanne Kappler, Fort Jackson Leader Newspaper: pages 173, 175

AP Photo/Carolyn Kaster: pages 179 (top left), 196 (bottom), 212

ICHIRO KATAKAI/a. collection RF/amanaimages/Corbis: page 56 (spiral notebook image)

Official White House Photo by Chuck Kennedy: pages 125, 172, 185 (left), 188

Chris Kirby: page 187 (bottom)

Ellen Kirby: pages 94 (right), 95 (left)

Eriko Koga/Digital Vision/Getty Images: page 248 (middle right)

Eddie Gehman Kohan: page 126 (top left)

Brooks Kraft/Corbis: pages 11, 32

Ken Krug: pages 33 (top), 63, 70–71, 108–109, 152–153, 204–205

SAUL LOEB/AFP/Getty Images: page 143 (bottom)

Rita Maas/ The Image Bank/ Getty

Images: page 239 (center)

Regine Mahaux/ Cultura RF/Getty Images: page 219 (center)

Kathryn McKenzie: page 139 (top left)

Judy McLin: page 187 (top)

Win McNamee/Getty Images: page 102 (right)

Gabriela Medina/Blend Images/ Getty Images: page 249 (top)

Doug Mills/The New York Times: page 33 (bottom)

Minnesota Historical Society/ CORBIS: page 29 (left)

AP Photo/Pablo Martinez Monsivais: pages 131, 198

Tracy Tomchik Nyszczot: page 134 (right)

Personal photos of the First Lady: pages 14, 15 (all)

Scott Olson/Getty Images: page 146

W. Pack / US National Archives and Records Administration: page 176

PEMCO Webster & Stevens Collection, Museum of History & Industry: page 101 (top)

Doug Pensinger /Allsport: page 200

PRNewsFoto/Welch's, Mary Plotts: page 126 (top right)

Martin Poole/ Getty Images: page 127 (right)

Chris J. Price/Getty Images: page 51 (bottom center)

Jason Reed/Reuters/Corbis: page 10

Rex Features via AP Images: pages 41 (top right), 48

MICHAEL REYNOLDS/epa/ Corbis: pages 57 (all), 203

PAUL J. RICHARDS/AFP/Getty Images: pages 46 (top), 126 (bottom right)

JEWEL SAMAD/AFP/Getty Images: page 184

Garra Schluter, Assistant Supervisor, Nutrition Services Bend LaPine Schools: page 189 (left)

INDEX

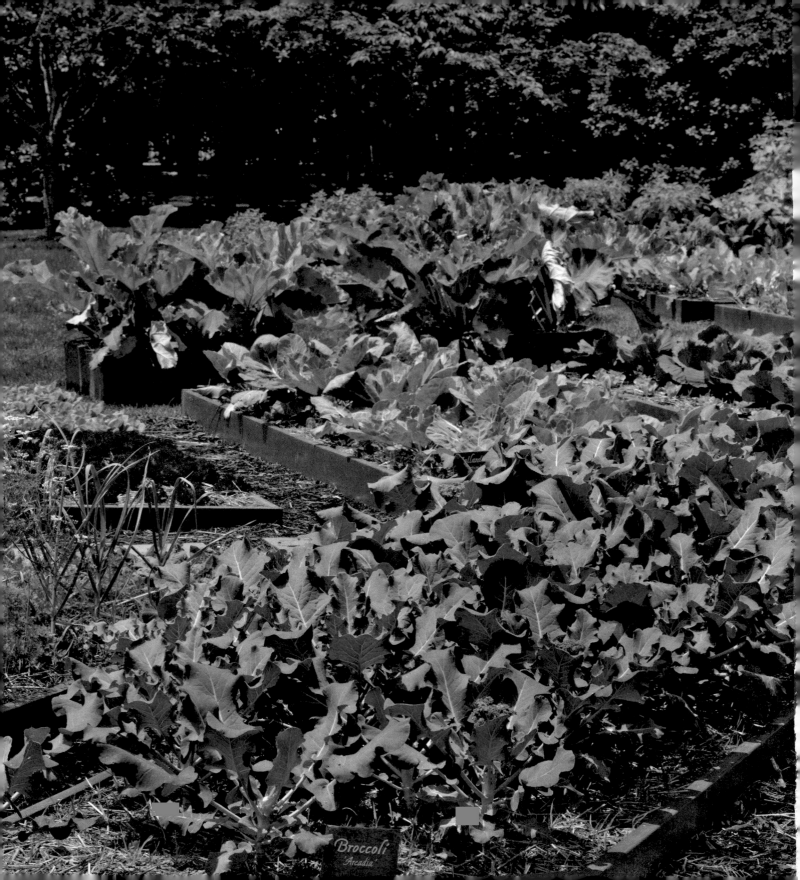